Synergy

The Unique Relationship Between Nurses and Patients

The AACN Synergy Model for Patient Care

Books Published by the Honor Society of Nursing, Sigma Theta Tau International

Synergy: The Unique Relationship Between Nurses and Patients, Martha A.Q. Curley, 2007.

Nursing Without Borders: Values, Wisdom, Success Markers, Sharon M. Weinstein and Ann Marie T. Brooks, 2007.

Johns Hopkins Evidence-Based Practice Model and Guidelines, Robin Newhouse, Sandra Dearholt, Stephanie Poe, Linda Pugh, and Kathleen White, 2007.

Conversations With Leaders: Frank Talk From Nurses (and Others) on the Front Lines of Leadership, Tine Hansen-Turton, Susan Sherman, Vernice Ferguson, 2007.

Pivotal Moments in Nursing: Leaders Who Changed the Path of a Profession, Beth Houser and Kathy Player, 2004 (Volume I) and 2007 (Volume II).

Shared Legacy, Shared Vision: The W. K. Kellogg Foundation and the Nursing Profession, Joan E. Lynaugh, Helen Grace, Gloria R. Smith, Roseni Sena, María Mercedes Dur·n de Villalobos, and Mary Malehloka Hlalele, 2007.

Daily Miracles: Stories and Practices of Humanity and Excellence in Health Care, Alan Briskin and Jan Boller, 2006.

A Daybook for Nurse Leaders and Mentors. Sigma Theta Tau International, 2006.

When Parents Say No: Religious and Cultural Influences on Pediatric Healthcare Treatment, Luanne Linnard-Palmer, 2006.

Healthy Places, Healthy People: A Handbook for Culturally Competent Community Nursing Practice, Melanie C. Dreher, Dolores Shapiro, and Micheline Asselin, 2006.

The HeART of Nursing: Expressions of Creative Art in Nursing, Second Edition, M. Cecilia Wendler, 2005.

Reflecting on 30 Years of Nursing Leadership: 1975-2005, Sr. Rosemary Donley, 2005

Technological Competency as Caring in Nursing, Rozzano Locsin, 2005.

Making a Difference: Stories from the Point of Care, Volume I, Sharon Hudacek, 2005.

A Daybook for Nurses: Making a Difference Each Day, Sharon Hudacek, 2004.

Making a Difference: Stories from the Point of Care, Volume II, Sharon Hudacek, 2004.

Building and Managing a Career in Nursing: Strategies for Advancing Your Career, Terry Miller, 2003.

Collaboration for the Promotion of Nursing, LeAlice Briggs, Sonna Ehrlich Merk, and Barbara Mitchell, 2003.

Ordinary People, Extraordinary Lives: The Stories of Nurses, Carolyn Smeltzer and Frances Vlasses, 2003.

Stories of Family Caregiving: Reconsideration of Theory, Literature, and Life, Suzanne Poirier and Lioness Ayres, 2002.

As We See Ourselves: Jewish Women in Nursing, Evelyn Benson, 2001.

Cadet Nurse Stories: The Call for and Response of Women During World War II, Thelma Robinson and Paulie Perry, 2001.

Creating Responsive Solutions to Healthcare Change, Cynthia McCullough, 2001.

The Language of Nursing Theory and Metatheory, Imogene King and Jacqueline Fawcett, 1997.

nurseAdvance Collection. (Topic-specific collections of honor society published journal articles.) Topics are: Cardiovascular Nursing; Cultural Diversity in Nursing; Disaster, Trauma, and Emergency Nursing; Ethical and Legal Issues in Nursing; Genomics in Nursing and Healthcare; Gerontological Nursing; Health Promotion in Nursing; Implementing Evidence-Based Nursing; Leadership and Mentoring in Nursing; Maternal Health Nursing; Oncology Nursing; Pain Management in Nursing; Pediatric Nursing; Psychiatric-Mental Health Nursing; Public, Environmental, and Community Health Nursing; and Women's Health Nursing; 2007.

To order any of these books, visit Nursing Knowledge International's Web site at **www.nursingknowledge.org/stti/ books**. Nursing Knowledge International is the honor society's sales and distribution division. You may also call 1.888.NKI.4.YOU (U.S. and Canada) or +1.317.634.8171 (Outside U.S. and Canada) to place an order.

Synergy

The Unique Relationship Between Nurses and Patients

The AACN Synergy Model for Patient Care

Martha A.Q. Curley, RN, PhD, FAAN

Sigma Theta Tau International
Honor Society of Nursing®

AMERICAN
ASSOCIATION
of CRITICAL-CARE
NURSES

Sigma Theta Tau International

Editor-in-Chief: Jeff Burnham
Acquisitions Editor: Cynthia Saver, RN, MS
Development Editor: Carla Hall
Copy Editor: Michelle Lilly
Editorial Team: Jane Palmer and Melody Jones
Indexer: Julie Bess

Cover Design by: Gary Adair
Interior Design and Page Composition by: Rebecca Harmon

Printed in the United States of America

Printing and Binding by Printing Partners, Indianapolis, Indiana, USA.

Sigma Theta Tau International
550 West North Street
Indianapolis, IN 46202

Visit our Web site at **www.nursingsociety.org** and go to the "Publications" link for more information about our books or other publications.

ISBN-10: 1-930538-51-0

ISBN-13: 978-1-930538-51-1

Library of Congress Cataloging-in-Publication Data

Synergy : the unique relationship between nurses and patients / [edited by] Martha A.Q. Curley.
         p. ; cm.
    Includes bibliographical references.
      ISBN 978-1-930538-51-1
   1. Nurse and patient. 2. Nursing models. I. Curley, Martha A. Q., 1952- II. Sigma Theta Tau International. III. American Association of Critical-Care Nurses.
      [DNLM: 1. Nursing Care--methods. 2. Models, Nursing. 3. Nurse-Patient Relations. 4. Patient Care Management--methods. WY 100 S992 2007]

RT86.3.S96 2007
610.73'0699--dc22

                                                          2007039990

07   08   09   10   11   /   5   4   3   2   1

Dedication

For my father, Angelo M. Quatrano (1925-2007)

Acknowledgments

The author and publisher join the American Association of Critical-Care Nurses and the AACN Certification Corporation in offering deep gratitude to the countless individuals and organizations who have made this book possible. Their creativity, wisdom, dedication, and enthusiasm ensured its success at every step. From development of the AACN Synergy Model for Patient Care through implementation in critical care credentialing, patient care, and nursing education, and now this tangible presentation of those experiences—without all these people, the results would assuredly have been very different.

About the Author

DR. CURLEY received her nursing diploma from Springfield Hospital School of Nursing, Springfield, Massachusetts. She received her bachelor's degree from the University of Massachusetts, Amherst, and her master's in pediatric acute care nursing from Yale University. She was awarded her PhD in 1997 from Boston College. She is currently an associate professor of nursing at the University of Pennsylvania School of Nursing. Dr. Curley is also a nurse scientist in critical care and cardiovascular nursing at Children's Hospital Boston and holds an appointment as lecturer-part time in anesthesia at Harvard Medical School.

Dr. Curley provided consistent leadership to a team of experts in developing the Synergy Model for Patient Care for the AACN Certification Corporation, the credentialing arm of the American Association of Critical-Care Nurses. The Synergy Model has been implemented for models of care delivery in practice environments and for certification exams and for curriculum in schools of nursing.

Dr. Curley has achieved wide recognition for her work related to clinical management of critically ill infants and children and their families, and also for her contributions to the field of pediatric critical care nursing. Her research focus has been on interventional studies to support parent needs and priorities in the pediatric intensive care unit, instrument development studies to provide clinicians with better tools to assess patient status and risk, and multi-site clinical trials to generate new knowledge in the care of critically ill pediatric patients.

Contributing Authors

JoAnn Grif Alspach, RN, MSN, EdD, FAAN (Chapter 12)

Dr. Alspach received her BSN and MSN in cardiovascular nursing from The Catholic University of America in Washington, DC, USA, and her doctorate in adult and continuing education from the University of Maryland, College Park. She has published 27 books and more than 120 journal articles and has lectured nationally and internationally in the areas of staff development, preceptor preparation, competency-based education, and critical care nursing. She is editor of the American Association of Critical-Care Nurses' *Core Curriculum for Critical Care Nursing*, as well as the *AACN Certification & Core Review for High Acuity and Critical Care*. She also serves as editor of *Critical Care Nurse* journal.

Linda E. Berlin, DrPH, RNC (Chapter 15)

Dr. Berlin is a principal with Berlin Sechrist Associates, a research consulting firm in Irvine, California, and Washington, DC, USA, that completed the Synergy Model scholarly critique process for the AACN Certification Corporation. She received a diploma in nursing from General Hospital (Rochester, New York), a BSN from the University of Arizona, a nurse practitioner certificate and MS from Albany Medical College, and a DrPH from the Johns Hopkins Bloomberg School of Public Health. Dr. Berlin has held faculty and/or clinical positions at Albany Medical College, Harvard School of Public Health, Massachusetts General Hospital, and The Johns Hopkins School of Medicine. She is a national authority on nursing and health workforce data.

Dora Bradley, PhD, RN-BC (Chapter 9)

Dr. Bradley is vice president of nursing professional development for Baylor Health Care System in Texas. She earned a baccalaureate from Oklahoma Baptist University, a master's from the University of Oklahoma, and a PhD in nursing science from the University of South Carolina. She is noted for her expertise in competency validation, program evaluation, and outcome measurement. Dr. Bradley became familiar with the Synergy Model when she was developing position descriptions for staff nurses and clinical nurse specialists. The model's relevance to actual practice, coupled with a focus on nursing outcomes and safe passage, was the catalyst for development of Baylor's Professional Nursing Practice Model and ASPIRE.

Barbara Brewer, PhD, RN, MLS, MBA (Chapter 16)

Dr. Brewer is director of professional practice at John C. Lincoln North Mountain Hospital in Phoenix, Arizona, USA. She became involved with the Synergy Model in her previous position as vice president of quality for Clarian Health in Indianapolis, Indiana. She holds adjunct faculty positions at The University of Arizona College of Nursing and Arizona State University College of Nursing and Healthcare Innovation. Dr. Brewer is a Magnet appraiser for the American Nurses Credentialing Center. She earned a BSN from the University of Rhode Island, an MA in liberal studies from Wesleyan University, an MSN from Yale University, an MBA from Columbia University, and a PhD in clinical nursing research from The University of Arizona.

Melanie Cline, MSN, RN (Chapter 7)

Ms. Cline is director of the pediatric specialty care center at Riley Hospital for Children, Clarian Health in Indianapolis, Indiana. She has been a leader in the development of the Clarian Synergy Professional Practice model, collaborating with Dr. Martha A. Q. Curley and the American Association of Critical-Care Nurses as one of the primary authors of the job documents and leader of the development of the patient side of the model. She has served as a consultant on behalf of Clarian to assist other systems in developing the Synergy model in other institutions. She earned her BSN from Purdue University and her MSN from Indiana University.

Marilyn Cox, MSN, RN (Chapter 7)

Ms. Cox is the senior vice president for nursing and patient care services at Riley Hospital for Children, part of the Clarian Health system in Indianapolis, Indiana. Ms. Cox earned both her baccalaureate and master's degree in nursing from the University of Oklahoma. She has served in nursing administrative positions for the past 29 years As the executive sponsor for the development of the Synergy Model for the Clarian system, she is responsible for the oversight and guidance of the model's application within the system. Ms. Cox is a Wharton Nursing Fellow and was recently selected for the HRET Safety Fellowship and completed this intensive course of study and project related to patient safety in 2007.

John F. Dixon, MSN, RN, CNA, BC (Chapter 9)

Mr. Dixon is a nurse researcher and nursing leadership/management consultant for the Center for Nursing Education and Research at Baylor University Medical Center in Dallas, Texas, USA. He earned a BA from Jacksonville University, a BSN from Florida State University, and an MSN from the University of Texas at Arlington. He is currently enrolled in the PhD in nursing program at the University of Texas at Arlington. Mr. Dixon has been an advocate of AACN's Synergy Model for Patient Care and AACN's Healthy Work Environment Standards, and has worked on methods of translation and dissemination for various facets of practice and operations. He was the primary designer for Baylor Health Care System's Professional Nursing Practice Model.

Sandra Greenberg, PhD (Chapter 14)

Dr. Greenberg is vice president for research and development at Professional Examination Services, a non-profit organization whose mission is to benefit the public good by promoting the understanding and use of sound credentialing practices in professions and occupations. She received her PhD in special education from Yeshiva University. She has coordinated numerous national and international job analysis studies of professions, conducted audits of existing certification programs, and provided consultative services to organizations regarding the development of new certification programs. She has developed outcomes-based and video-based assessments for physicians and performance assessments for allied health personnel.

Sonya R. Hardin, RN, PhD, CCRN, APRN-BC (Chapter 10)

Dr. Hardin received her PhD from the University of Colorado Health Sciences Center, MSN and BSN from the University of North Carolina at Charlotte, and MSN/MHA from Pfeiffer University. She completed postdoctoral work at the University of North Carolina at Chapel Hill. She is an associate professor in the School of Nursing at the University of North Carolina at Charlotte. Dr. Hardin has served on several task forces for the American Association of Critical-Care Nurses, including those focused on development of the Synergy Model, study of practice, and standard of practice. She is coauthor of *Synergy for Clinical Excellence: The AACN Synergy Model for Patient Care* and *Critical Care Nursing: Optimal Patient Outcomes*. Her research focuses on quality of life issues for heart failure patients.

Carol Hartigan, RN, BSN, MA (Chapter 6)

Ms. Hartigan serves on the national staff of the American Association of Critical-Care Nurses as certification strategist for the AACN Certification Corporation, the association's credentialing arm. Ms. Hartigan has served on the board of directors of the National Organization of Competency Assurance, as NCLEX contract manager for the National Council of State Boards of Nursing, and associate executive director of the Missouri State Board of Nursing. She was an instructor of nursing at Missouri Western State College and critical care educator at Methodist Medical Center in St. Joseph, Missouri. A nursing graduate of Missouri Western State College and Northwest Missouri State University, Ms. Hartigan received her master's degree in adult and continuing education from the University of Missouri-Kansas City.

Carolyn Hayes, RN, PhD (Chapter 8)

Dr. Hayes is a nursing director at the Dana-Farber Cancer Institute (DFCI) and Brigham and Women's Hospital (BWH) in Boston, Massachusetts, USA. She is accountable for inpatient nursing and clinical services on seven BWH hematology/oncology/bone marrow transplantation patient-care areas and continuum of care programs at DFCI. Dr. Hayes received her BSN from Georgetown University, her MS from the University of Illinois at Chicago, and her PhD from Boston College. She completed a post-master's fellowship in administration at University of Chicago Hospitals and a postdoctoral fellowship in medical ethics at Harvard Medical School. Her clinical work, teaching, writing, and research have focused on clinical ethics, end-of-life decision making, nursing administration, and integrative therapies.

Kimmith M. Jones, RN, MS, CCNS (Chapter 5)

Kimmith Jones is the advanced practice nurse/clinical nurse specialist for Critical Care Services at Sinai Hospital of Baltimore. He received his MSN from the University of Maryland with a focus in trauma/critical care. He is a past board member and chairperson of the AACN Certification Corporation. During his time on the board of directors, he was involved with the development of the Synergy Model.

Maureen Leonardo, MN, RN, CNE, CRNP, BC (Chapter 11)

Ms. Leonardo, associate professor of nursing at Duquesne University in Pittsburgh, Pennsylvania, earned her BSN from Indiana University of Pennsylvania and her MSN from the University of Pittsburgh. She has been a leader and driving force in the implementation of the AACN Synergy Model of Patient Care in the educational program. Ms. Leonardo is a strong community advocate and assists senior citizens within the community in maintaining their health and independence through the School of Nursing's Nurse Managed Wellness Centers. She is the recipient of the Dean's Award for Teaching Excellence and was honored as a 2007 Cameo of Caring recipient for the annual Pittsburgh-wide celebration of nurses.

Anne Micheli, RN, MSN (Chapter 3)

Ms. Micheli, director of perioperative and allied programs for nursing and patient services with Children's Hospital Boston, earned her BSN from Northeastern University in Boston, Massachusetts, and her MSN from Boston University. She was an original member of the Children's Professional Advancement Committee and has been involved with development, implementation, and evaluation of the Professional Advancement Program. Ms. Micheli has served in many leadership roles throughout her career and is a longtime advocate for establishment of a strong shared governance model with her departments and throughout the hospital. In 2005, she won the New England ADVANCE for Nurses Best Nurse Leaders award in the category of Leading by Example.

Patricia A. Moloney-Harmon, RN, MS, CCNS, CCRN, FAAN (Chapter 5)

Patricia Moloney-Harmon is an advanced practice nurse/clinical nurse specialist for children's services at Sinai Hospital of Baltimore. She provides consultation to the nursing staff regarding pediatric critical care and emergency issues. She has coordinated numerous patient safety initiatives throughout the institution, including reduction in medication errors. She received her BSN and MSN with a focus on trauma/critical care from the University of Maryland. She is a past board member and chairperson of the AACN Certification Corporation. During her time on the board of directors, she was involved with the development of the Synergy Model.

Patricia M. Muenzen, MA (Chapter 14)

Ms. Muenzen is director of research programs at Professional Examination Services, a non-profit organization whose mission is to benefit the public good by promoting the understanding and use of sound credentialing practices in professions and occupations. She received her MA degree in psychology from Stony Brook University. She has conducted numerous studies related to competencies, knowledge, and skills underlying the practice of professions and has served for several years on the research committee for the American Board of Nursing Specialties.

Christine M. Pacini, PhD, RN (Chapter 13)

Dr. Pacini is director of the Center for Professional Development, Research and Innovation for the University of Michigan Health System. She has used the Synergy Model to create a curriculum that supports the advancement of clinical nurses by developing the skills and competencies embedded within the nurse characteristics. Dr. Pacini received her PhD in nursing with a cognate in neuroscience from the University of Michigan. She earned an MSN from Wayne State University, a BSN from Mercy College of Detroit, and a BA from the University of Detroit. Previously, she served as director of education at Clarian Health, associate dean and chairperson of the McAuley School of Nursing at the University of Detroit Mercy, and associate administrator for nursing development and research at Henry Ford Hospital.

Stephanie Packard, RN, ADN (Chapter 4)

Ms. Packard is a level III staff nurse in the neonatal intensive care unit at Children's Hospital Boston in Massachusetts. She is the NICU performance improvement coordinator. She co-chairs the Hospital Professional Advancement Committee and the Professional Advancement Board of Review. She holds an associate's degree in nursing from Central Maine Medical Center School of Nursing.

Kevin Reed, MSN, RN, CNA-BC, CPHQ (Chapter 7)

Mr. Reed is the director of clinical operations for adult critical care services and the neurosciences at Methodist Hospital/Clarian Health in Indianapolis, Indiana. He is also the current chairman of the board of AACN Certification Corporation. Mr. Reed received his BSN from Ball State University in 1983 and his MSN in administration from Indiana University School of Nursing in 1993. He has more than 20 years experience in various critical care nursing leadership positions. He has been a strong supporter of the application of the Synergy Model in the clinical practice environment.

Karen R. Sechrist, PhD, RN, FAAN (Chapter 15)

Dr. Sechrist is a principal and research specialist with Berlin Sechrist Associates, a contract research and research-related projects group located in Irvine, California, and Washington, DC. AACN Certification Corporation contracted with Berlin Sechrist Associates to complete the Synergy Model scholarly critique process. She received an Associate in Arts in nursing from Pasadena City College, a Bachelor of Science in Nursing from Wheaton College, a Master of Science in Nursing from DePaul University, and a PhD in higher education from the University of Pittsburgh. Dr. Sechrist held graduate teaching and research positions in nursing in three major universities and was director of research for the American Association of Critical-Care Nurses prior to joining Berlin Sechrist Associates.

I. Leon Smith, PhD (Chapter 14)

Dr. Smith is president and chief executive officer of Professional Examination Services, a non-profit organization whose mission is to benefit the public good by promoting the understanding and use of sound credentialing practices in professions and occupations. He received his PhD in educational psychology from the State University of New York at Buffalo. He has presented papers and published widely on topics related to competency assessment in credentialing and transitioning assessments from paper-and-pencil to computer-based delivery. Dr. Smith has also served as a commissioner for the National Commission for Certifying Agencies—an organization that accredits certification programs meeting its standards—and co-chaired a commission task force charged with reviewing and revising the commission's accreditation standards. In 2005, he received the organization's leadership award for his contributions to the field of certification.

Eileen Zungolo, EdD, RN, CNE, FAAN (Chapter 11)

Dr. Zungolo is a former Fulbright Scholar and recipient of the Leader of Leaders Award from the National Student Nurses' Association in 2005, and is dean and professor of nursing at Duquesne University in Pittsburgh, Pennsylvania. Originally educated at St. Francis Hospital School of Nursing, she earned her bachelor's, master's, and doctoral degrees from Teachers College, Columbia University. Her career includes a number of years in nursing practice in acute care and pediatrics. For the last 30 years, she has been a dedicated nurse educator. Dr. Zungolo was president of the National League for Nursing from 2001-03. She was among the inaugural group to earn certification as a nurse educator and is a fellow in the American Academy of Nursing and the Academy of Nursing Education.

Table of Contents

Foreword

The basic premise of the Synergy Model is simple, elegant, and historically embedded in the practice of nursing.
—Martha A. Q. Curley, RN, PhD, FAAN

The AACN Synergy Model for Patient Care represents the enduring contribution of some of critical care nursing's brightest and most insightful thought leaders. The model is predicated on Virginia Henderson's intuitively basic premise about the nurse-patient relationship: Nurses assist in "the performance of those activities … that [the patient] would perform unaided if [he or she] had the necessary strength, will, or knowledge" (Henderson, 1960). The Synergy Model expands and focuses Henderson's premise by recognizing that nurses' competencies are, in fact, universally driven by what patients and their families need.

It is very appropriate that Martha A. Q. Curley is this book's editor and contributor, since her name is often associated with the AACN Synergy Model for Patient Care. As a member of the expert panel that developed the model, Dr. Curley examined its potential in her doctoral research, wrote the seminal *American Journal of Critical Care* article describing the model, and championed its earliest use in patient care at Children's Hospital Boston.

Over the years, visionary leaders have adopted the model in varying degrees in their individual practices, in discrete patient-care environments, and most recently, across entire health systems. In 2001, Dr. Karlene Kerfoot and nurse leaders at Clarian Health recognized the model's inherent power, selecting it as the patient-care model for this 1,200-bed health system that is Indiana's largest. Theirs is the first system-wide implementation of the Synergy Model. I joined Clarian's team as an advanced practice nurse in 2004 and have had the privilege of experiencing firsthand how the model can serve as a catalyst for excellent professional practice and drive a health-care organization's effort to ensure safe and reliable care for patients and families. Colleagues at Baylor Health Care System in Dallas are now successfully doing the same.

Educators such as Dr. Sonya Hardin have adopted the Synergy Model as a framework for effective teaching strategies with undergraduate nursing students. In 2002, Dr. Eileen Zungolo and her colleagues recognized the Synergy Model's potential as the framework for an academic curriculum, selecting the model to guide the baccalaureate and master's nursing programs at Duquesne University.

The American Association of Critical-Care Nurses designated Clarian Health Partners as its clinical incubator for the model and Duquesne University School of Nursing as its academic incubator.

AACN applauds the contributions to excellent patient care described in this landmark book. We commend Dr. Curley for her passionate enthusiasm in support of the Synergy Model. And we thank the Honor Society of Nursing, Sigma Theta Tau International for its collaboration in making publication possible.

–M. David Hanson, RN, MSN, CCRN, CNS
President, 2007-08
American Association of Critical-Care Nurses

Preface

Workforce shortages and vast health-care changes continue to focus the attention of hospitals on review and modification of the way care is organized and delivered to patients. Central in this search for new and improved care delivery systems is the profession of nursing, which seeks to develop and advance a professional practice model. This search for new delivery system models and advancing the professionalism of nursing practice seems to be never ending—perhaps because the emphasis is often on change, which for many suggests the notion of doing something very different. As a result, the health-care system is sometimes blessed with creative approaches and at other times bogged down with the problem of "throwing the baby out with the bath water."

What is often overlooked in this search is that in defining a practice, there are significant elements that have stood the test of time no matter the multiple organizational and system changes that take place. These elements should become the focus of the challenge for creativity as well as thoughtfulness in responding to the never-ending process of change. In recent years, nurse researchers have provided increasing evidence to support the important clinical role of nurses in ensuring positive patient care outcomes. The centrality of nursing practice within the care delivery system and contributions of nurses, independent of those of others involved in care delivery, are demonstrated in the work of Linda Aiken and her research associates, as well as in the research of Peter Buerhaus, Jack Needleman, and—increasingly—that of others. Studies such as these have helped the field better understand that the context of nursing practice is an essential element in determining the possibilities of practice. This context is both internal and external. That is, the provider of care—the nurse—brings certain attributes, background, and competencies to the caregiving process. In addition, the nurse is influenced by the work environment, the resources available, and the organizational values of and understanding about clinical practice. Although most practice model experimentation is intended to be more efficient in the delivery of care and services, often there is also the desire to increase the professional aspects of care delivery by increasing nurse autonomy, decision-making, and collaboration with others in the development of expected outcomes. Yet, the field varies widely in the application of a professional practice model, calling for strong and sustained leadership efforts to advance the practice of nursing.

Most of us learned from Virginia Henderson's definition of nursing that the core of practice is the nurse-patient relationship. No matter the context—or the external environment—individual care planning by nurse professionals is a central need of patients and was viewed by Miss Henderson as the essence of nursing practice (1980). It is this relationship that is the underlying principle of a professional practice model. It is also this relationship that all other relationships stem from, including collaboration with physicians and other health professionals, with other nurse colleagues, and with families and other significant relationships. The participation of the nurse in decision-making, collaboration, and communication comes from the primary relationship of nurse and patient. So, as experimentation is undertaken with new roles, practice models, and other organizational redesign, the question that should remain at the core of the change process is: "How can we keep the nurse in a direct-care relationship with the patient?" By doing so, we recognize the time-honored nature of nursing practice, but we do more than that as well. We affirm the practice of our discipline, for there really is no practice, no knowing of the patient therapeutically, no understanding of the ongoing needs of this person within the context of his or her environment without such a relationship. Without this relationship, nursing becomes simply the carrying out of tasks and activities in virtually a void of essential information.

What is understood universally is that a practice is a web of values, behaviors, character, knowledge, and skill that is reworked, refined, and extended through generations. In other words, the essence of what it means to be a nurse does not change; it is the context, technology, social values, science, and economics that will change. What has not changed is that relationships and care are central to practice. Without a relationship—without *synergy* in other words—between the nurse and the patient, what the educated and professionally socialized nurse brings to the situation is absent. Care is not simply being nice. Rather, it is working with the other to achieve what is in the other's best interest—the helping notion embedded in Henderson's definition of nursing.

Thus, in spite of the significant system changes, it is important to stay aware of the time-honored nature of practice, of the foundation of practice, even though they may be periodically contemporized by the environment. Today, the important relationship of nurse and patient is spoken of as "knowing the patient" and is often referred to as the heart of nursing practice. It bears repeating: It is through the nurse-patient relationship that all other health-care relationships are developed and strengthened. The relationship between nurse and patient inevitably increases the amount of information the nurse has about patients, and thus improves communication by providing more relevant information to others and supporting the nurse's position of leadership and accountability for patient care.

One thing that we can count on for the future is the continuing search for innovation in the development of new practice models. Practice is linked to and shaped by the context in which it occurs, to the changing environment of health care and to the organizational, political, or professional policies that shape the systems of care delivery. The challenge, therefore, is in making the future practice models flexible enough to respond to the changing context of practice, while staying focused on the time-honored essence of nursing practice. The AACN Synergy Model for Patient Care exemplifies this relationship.

Joyce C. Clifford, RN, PhD, FAAN, is the president and CEO of The Institute for Nursing Healthcare Leadership (INHL) representing the Consortium of Harvard-Affiliated Nursing Services. She was senior vice president for nursing programs at CareGroup in Boston before the establishment of INHL. She was vice president and nurse-in-chief at Beth Israel Hospital in Boston, a position she held for more than 25 years, before the merger of Beth Israel and Deaconess hospitals. Dr. Clifford is an established author and consultant on the subject of organizational restructuring and the development of a professional practice model.

The Synergy Model: From Theory to Practice

Martha A.Q. Curley, RN, PhD, FAAN

This is an exciting time for the profession of nursing. Having withstood a decade or more of health-care restructuring and re-engineering, nurses are building a much-needed evidence base to link nursing care to positive patient outcomes and to safer care environments. Responding to unprecedented nursing shortages, many employers offer nurses significant incentives and work hard to keep experienced nurses within their systems by acknowledging the need to provide ongoing clinical support and a professional practice milieu.

In this environment focused on nurse recruitment and best practices, the voices rising up from the nursing profession must be universally clear on what stellar nursing care is and what the expected patient and system outcomes are when this kind of care is practiced. Patients and families today are informed consumers and seek care from nurses in whom they can establish immediate trust. These nurses must be knowledgeable, caring, and savvy clinicians. Health-care delivery models must be designed so patients and families know their nurses and nurses know their patients.

This health-care environment presents a unique opportunity for the nursing profession—an opportunity to thoroughly describe nursing practice and to test new models of care delivery. Nurses must have a clear understanding of what they do, what their relationships are to patients and families, and what effects they have on patient outcomes. Nursing cannot be effectively measured and directly linked to patient outcomes until nurses can easily describe their practice.

What Nurses Do

The credentialing arm of the American Association of Critical-Care Nurses (AACN) began work on the AACN Synergy Model for Patient Care™ more than a decade ago to better explain critical care nursing practice. At the time, the AACN Certification Corporation was planning a third validation study to ensure that the CCRN® credential accurately reflected contemporary critical care nursing practice. Simply stated, the Synergy Model is a conceptual framework describing a patient-nurse relationship that acknowledges the primary importance of nursing care based on the needs of patients and their families. The fundamental premise of the Synergy Model is that patients' characteristics drive nurse competencies. When patient characteristics and nurse competencies are in synergy, optimal patient outcomes are more likely to occur (see Figure 1.1). Soon after its publication, the Synergy Model crossed traditional subspecialty boundaries and reverberated as a relevant model for patient care wherever patients and nurses were found.

Synergy Model

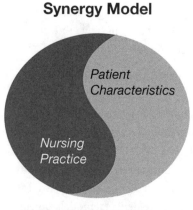

Optimal Patient Outcomes

Figure 1.1. The Synergy Model
Adapted with permission. (Curley, 1998).

Conceptual models are important because they help illuminate what is essential or relevant to a discipline. Visintainer (1986) used an analogy of maps to identify what is important or relevant to a discipline. For example, a collection of maps describes a region of the world and can describe different aspects of that region—weather, air currents, temperature, rainfall, road and air traffic control, and geological features. While all maps accurately describe the region, which map is best depends on the information needed or the question being asked. Similarly, while many wonderful conceptual models describe nursing, the Synergy Model specifically describes relevant aspects of nurse-patient, nurse-nurse, and nurse-system relationships.

Many health-care systems use a conceptual framework to unify their thinking around nursing practice within their facility. The Synergy Model is a practical and intuitive framework that resonates with nurses from varying subspecialties and levels of expertise, and roles ranging from staff nurse to chief nurse executive. The Synergy Model resonates with clinicians because it describes what nurses do based on the primacy of patients and optimal nurse-patient relationships. The synergy that occurs within the relationship is unique to the profession and mutual in effect as it not only benefits patients, but it calls attention to therapeutic patient-nurse relationships that serve to sustain nurses within the profession. Specifically, reciprocal nurse-patient/family relationships carry the potential for providing an enormous source of professional satisfaction for nurses (Curley, 1997).

The basic premise of the Synergy Model is simple, elegant, and historically embedded in the practice of nursing. Nurses have always done what patients needed and were unable to do for themselves. Virginia Henderson (1960) described the nurse-patient relationship as:

> She [the nurse] must, in a sense, "get inside the skin" of each of her patients
> in order to know what he needs. She is temporarily the consciousness of
> the unconscious, the love of life for the suicidal, the leg of the amputee, the
> eyes of the newly blind, a means of locomotion for the infant, knowledge
> and confidence for the young mother, the "mouthpiece" for those too weak
> or withdrawn to speak, and so on.

In these powerful words, written more than half a century ago, nurses do what patients and families need for them to do. Henderson goes on to say:

> Nursing is primarily assisting the individual (sick or well) in the performance
> of those activities contributing to health, or his recovery (or to a peaceful
> death) that he would perform unaided if he had the necessary strength, will,
> or knowledge. It is likewise the unique contribution of Nursing to help the
> individual to be independent of such assistance as soon as possible.

So, while nurses base their practice on patient needs, their goal is to help the patient and family become functionally independent. More recently, the *"provision of a caring relationship that facilitates health and healing"* was acknowledged by the American Nurses Association (2003a) as an essential feature of contemporary nursing practice. The essence of nursing is the primacy of patients and doing what patients and their families need through caring relationships that facilitate healing. The Synergy Model describes these fundamental elements of nursing.

The Synergy Model describes a cluster of personal characteristics that each patient and family bring to a health-care situation. The eight patient characteristics, which span a continuum of health to illness, are stability, complexity, vulnerability, predictability, resiliency, participation in decision-making, participation in care, and resource availability. Nursing competencies, derived from the needs of patients, are also described in terms of essential continuums. The Synergy Model describes eight nurse dimensions of nursing practice that span the continuum from competent to expert: clinical judgment, clinical inquiry, caring practices, response to diversity, advocacy/moral agency, facilitation of learning, collaboration, and systems thinking. These competencies reflect a dynamic integration of knowledge, skills, experience, and attitudes needed to meet patient needs and optimize patient outcomes. In this model, optimal patient outcomes result when patient characteristics and nurse competencies synergize. Optimal outcomes are what patients themselves (or people significant to patients) define as important. Three levels of outcomes are described in the Synergy Model: patient/family-level, unit-level, and system-level.

Moving the Synergy Model Into Clinical Practice

Applying the Synergy Model to clinical practice brings both the work of nursing and the model to life. The Synergy Model can be used to describe patient needs, nurse competencies, models of care, and outcome indicators that derive from the nurse-patient relationship.

Patient Needs

Nurses can use the Synergy Model to better describe: (1) individual patient needs during nurse-to-nurse report, and (2) a group of patient needs using second generation "acuity" or "needs" scoring systems.

Nurse-to-Nurse Report

Every day, every shift, nurses tell the story of the patient and his or her family to another nurse during nurse-to-nurse sign-out or shift change so that care can continue as smoothly as possible. Though unit-specific in format, nurse-to-nurse sign-outs usually entail a statement of the patient's problem, past medical history, review of systems, current orders, team members, social supports, and a heads-up to the patient's likes and dislikes (see Box 1.1). Documentation systems, sometimes computerized, are used to organize sign-out information.

Optimally, the sign-out also provides an opportunity for nurse-to-nurse coaching and mentoring of the salience of the patient's trajectory of illness. Helping the oncoming nurse benefit from what was learned about the patient and family augments the oncoming nurse's capacity to know the patient. Knowing the patient is a caring practice that includes knowing the patient and family as individuals and having an in-depth knowledge of their typical response (Tanner, Benner, Chesla, & Gordon, 1993). Knowing the patient refers to how the nurse understands the patient, grasps the meaning of the situation for the patient, or recognizes the need for a particular intervention. Knowing the patient requires clinical judgment and creates possibility for advocacy that limits patient vulnerability and prevents iatrogenic injury. The eight patient dimensions of the Synergy Model can then be used to help communicate nurse knowledge of the patient and family.

For example, review Ann's sign-out report in Box 1.1. Ann is a 5-year-old female post cardiopulmonary arrest of unclear etiology. Her sign-out describes her as unstable, complex, vulnerable, unpredictable, resilient—having survived a full cardiopulmonary arrest—with an engaged family who is actively participating in decision-making and care with adequate resource availability. Summarizing these eight characteristics during nurse-to-nurse sign-out provides a minimum data set describing Ann's needs and also creates "teachable" moments for the coaching and mentoring of less experienced colleagues. When considering Ann's needs, the charge nurse would assign a proficient pediatric critical care nurse. The clinical nurse specialist (CNS) would probably start at Ann's bedside when making rounds.

Box 1.1. Pediatric Critical Care Patient Profile

Ann is a 5-year-old girl who suffered a full cardiopulmonary arrest yesterday in the emergency department (ED) after presenting in shock after a 2-day history of fever, vomiting, and abdominal pain. She has a positive medical history—hospitalized 2.5 years ago with idiopathic dilated cardiomyopathy that responded well to therapy. She was off all medications (digoxin, diuretics, and enalapril) and was considered to be in excellent health 2 weeks before in cardiology clinic.

Pre-arrest in the ED, she was poorly perfused and lethargic but able to respond appropriately. Quick look echocardiogram (ECHO) revealed severe systolic left-ventricular (LV) dysfunction. Post-arrest, she was unable to sustain an adequate blood pressure with maximal conventional therapy, so she was emergently transferred to the intensive care unit (ICU) and placed on extracorporeal membrane oxygenation (ECMO).

The working diagnosis is profound cardiac failure of questionable etiology. The plan is to maintain ECMO support and consider cardiac transplantation if her neurological evaluation is reasonable.

She had an unstable night; the major problem has been bleeding from her ECMO cannula sites.

She was re-explored twice but continues with 80-100 mL of chest tube drainage per hour.

Blood bank has been able to keep up with her losses, providing continuous replacement of packed cells, 5% albumin, FFP, platelets, and cryoprecipitate.
She is on Amicar continuous infusion at 750 mg/hr (per ECMO protocol).

Review of Systems and Current Orders

Cardiopulmonary

She is on ECMO with an open chest and 3 transthoracic cannulas: 2 venous (1 RA & 1 LA) and 1 arterial return to the aorta.

She has an occlusive transparent dressing over her open chest.

Ann's skin is still pale and mottled; capillary refill is 4-5 sec; extremities are cool and she appears puffy; has periorbital edema.

Overnight, our goal has been to keep her MAPs around 70 mmHg, RAP <15 mmHg and LAP <10 mmHg by increasing ECMO flow as much as possible; with volume replacement; and by manipulating epinephrine, dopamine, and amrinone.

Because of inadequate venous cannula size, we've been unable to increase her flow more than 1.8 L/min. The cardiac surgeons would like to replace her RA cannula with a larger size later this morning.

We've kept up with her mediastinal drainage—replacing cc per cc. You have to stay on top of her 3 mediastinal drains because they clot easily.

Ann was initially hypotensive, with MAPs in the 50s, but she weaned off epinephrine by midnight then weaned to renal dose (2.5 mcg/kg/min) dopamine by 2 a.m. At 4 a.m. cardiology recommended that we start amrinone for afterload reduction; she's now on 5 mcg/kg/min—they also discussed nitroglycerin, which may be used later.

Ann has been in normal sinus rhythm/sinus tachycardia (NSR/ST) most of the night.

She did have a short period of ventricular fibrillation (VF) during her first exploration but easily converted to NSR with 20 joules using internal paddles.

After that we bolused her with Lidocaine 20mg, then started a Lidocaine drip at 20 mcg/kg/min.

She has had no spontaneous arrhythmias since; 06:00 Lidocaine level = 2.04. Given her contractility, they might want to discontinue this.

She has A&V wires in place; the pacemaker captures easily but we haven't needed it.

She is intubated with an oral 5.0 mm cuffed ET tube—cuff is down.

She is on 25/5, 0.6 F_IO_2 at a rate of 10; the high F_IO_2 is for coronary artery perfusion.

Breath sounds are equal with bilateral scattered rhonchi that clear somewhat after suctioning.

She was suctioned twice—last time was at 5 a.m. for a scant amount of thin white secretions.

Last set of gases: arterial 7.47/34/314/24/100% and mixed venous 7.42/40/42/25/79%.

Parameters have changed all night—check to see what is decided on rounds.

Hematology

Hct: 23.7; PT 16.2; Platelets 129K; Fibrinogen 187.

Heparin requirements have decreased overnight—ACTs currently 200.

Her evolving coagulopathy may be due to sepsis.

Infectious Disease

We're keeping her temperature at 95° fahrenheit (35° celsius) to decrease metabolic requirements.

Full cultures were sent yesterday—nothing preliminary thus far.

She is on triple antibiotic coverage.

Fluids, Electrolytes, and Nutrition

Maintenance fluids D5/0.25 NS with 10mEq KCL at 30 mL/hr

Potassium bolus x 2 for K^+ level of 3.0; Calcium gluconate bolus x 1 for Cal 8.9

06:00 labs: Na 147; K 3.2; Cl 94; TCO_2 32; BS 152; Ical 0.94; Cal 8.6; Phos 5.5; Mg 2.2; TP 5.8; Alb 2.8

Need to order TPN/Lipids today.

Neurological

Pupils are midposition with a sluggish response to both direct and consensual light—last dose of atropine received about 18 hours ago.

No cough, gag, corneals, or doll's eyes.

No spontaneous movement.

+ 4 thumb abduction to train-of-four stimulation—no pavulon since cannulation yesterday.

Her lowest pH during her arrest was 6.99.

Neurology will see her today (baseline: doing well in kindergarten).

Comfort: Receiving 1.5 mg/hr of morphine; may consider lorazepam q8hrs and midazolam prn.

Renal

BUN 48; creatinine 1.7

No urine output—foley irrigated with normal saline—bladder not palpable.

Bolus x 1 with furosemide without diuresis.

ICU attending mentioned a continuous furosemide infusion—check with renal.

Renal team will consult today—anticipate CVVH/dialysis via the ECMO circuit tomorrow.

Gastrointestinal

No bowel sounds; nasogastric tube (NGT) to suction; 100mL bilious Heme + drainage.

On ranitidine.

Skin

She has a jell pad under her occiput.

On an Effica CC bed at 5ft—no turns with open chest.

Ask the specialty bed company to send in their CNS for a bed adjustment.

Vascular access

She has more than adequate access.

Pressors and sedation are going into the circuit.

You can use the RA for blood products; LA is transduced.

She has a right double-lumen femoral.

She has a right radial A-line that draws well.

Social

Ann is 5 years old and is the third of four children. The other children are ages 11, 7, and 3 months. Parents are married and live together. Dad is a fireman and mom is a teacher but currently on maternity leave.

Parents are upset. Both are here and aware of her status. Both have seen her recently. They, especially Dad, can only stay at the bedside for a few minutes before they have to leave. Mom is able to ask questions and appears to be processing information. The other children are in their aunt's care—there is a large extended family.

Team

Dr. X is Ann's cardiologist; Dr. X is on for heart transplant; X is the on call nurse.

Dr. X is the cardiac surgeon; Dr. X is the fellow; Dr. X is the ICU physician; Dr. X is on for ECMO; Dr. X is on for neurology; and Dr. X is on for the renal team. Primary care physician is Dr. X, who appears to have a very good relationship with the parents.

Summary Statement

Ann is a 5-year-old female, status post cardiopulmonary arrest of unclear etiology. The team is hopeful that she has reversible single organ (cardiac) failure. If not reversible and only single system (no neurological sequelae), she will be listed for heart transplant. Ann is extremely sensitive to even slight physiological changes and requires moment-to-moment vigilant monitoring and reciprocal interventions to manage her tenuous status. Her medical team is very large, and it has been very difficult to develop and maintain one cohesive unifying plan. Ann's family is devastated, but everyone appears mutually supportive. The team has been communicating well with the family.

Acuity Scoring Systems

Historically, acuity scoring systems have been used to predict nurse-to-patient ratios on inpatient units. These systems typically include an inventory of tasks and the necessary amount of time required by nurses to accomplish each task. The patient's overall trajectory of illness, available nursing expertise, and the importance of continuity in nurse-patient relationships over an episode of illness are seldom taken into consideration (Curley & Hickey, 2006).

Doble, Curley, Hession-Laband, Marino, and Shaw (2000) described a project in which a group of nurse experts used the Synergy Model as the conceptual model to classify patient nursing needs based on the diagnosis related group (DRG), specifically the all patient refined DRG (APR-DRG) which levels DRGs by severity of illness and risk of mortality. First, data sheets for each level of each APR-DRG were created to demonstrate a profile of the patient group being categorized. Each data sheet reflected the hospital's most recent data—specifically, the number and name of the APR-DRG, levels 1 to 4, numbers of patients with that DRG over the span of a year, percentage of patients who were cared for in the ICU, percentage who died, associated primary diagnoses and secondary diagnoses, primary and secondary procedures, age group, and length-of-stay (LOS) average and range. In total, each profile provided a snapshot of the patients within the specific APR-DRG.

Using the Synergy Model allowed the nurse experts—one nurse from each clinical area—a common language to describe patient needs and the nursing competencies required by "an average patient on an average day" within each APR-DRG. The nurse experts first sorted each DRG data sheet into "low" and "high" categories relative to *patient char-*

acteristics. For example, the facilitator posed the following questions when reviewing each data sheet: How stable is this patient population? How vulnerable are the patients? How predictable is their course? How many services are typically involved with the population?

The experts then used the *nursing characteristics* to sort the "low" group into 3 clusters (1, 2, or 3) and the "high" group into 3 clusters (4, 5, or 6). For example, the experts would note: "Proficient clinical judgment is required; collaborative skills should be a priority because the teams are large, and well-honed systems savvy is necessary because of all the transition points involved in the patient's care." Including one nurse from each clinical area ensured that each diagnostic group was known to at least one nurse and built reliability into the process, as all expert nurses had to agree with each diagnostic group's final classification. An hour standard was then attached to each cluster level (1 though 6) to link how much nursing time was required to meet the needs of the typical patient within each APR-DRG.

Retrospectively, the difference between the projected patient needs per APR-DRG (cluster hours) and actual nursing hours worked on a unit was assessed for trends. (See Figure 1.2.) These unit-based reports plot the APR-DRG cluster hours (patient needs) and the total hours worked per day per unit per month. Note: the hours track well in April but not in May, when several additional nurses were on orientation. The grids can be subjectively validated by asking charge nurses to give their impression of staffing on each shift over the month's time. Differences in projections and subjective assessments can be attributed to the level of expertise of the nurses who constitute the hour standard.

Nurse Competencies

The nurse dimensions of the Synergy Model can be used to frame nursing competence within health-care organizations and professional certification. Articulating minimal competencies in all eight dimensions can form the basis of nursing job descriptions. Once the minimum is defined, articulating evolving expertise within each dimension and linking that evolution to levels of practice can form the basis of a professional advancement program (Czerwinski, Blastic, & Rice, 1999). Once the level of expertise is differentiated, the optimal balance of competent, proficient, and expert staff nurses on a unit can be determined based on the needs of the patient population served.

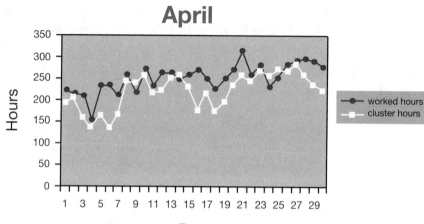

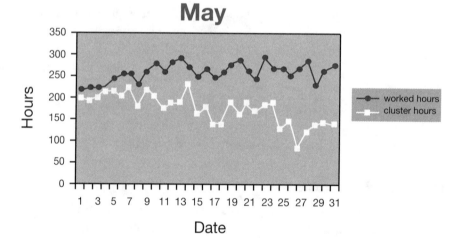

Figure 1.2.   Retrospective analysis comparing the total patient needs (per DRG) on a nursing unit (cluster hours) to the actual number of nurses' worked hours. Data appear matched in April but not matched in May (more nurse hours worked than required by patient needs per DRG).

Using the same conceptual model for all nursing job descriptions serves to highlight similarities and differences between nursing roles within complex organizations. While nurse practitioners and clinical nurse specialists are each considered advanced practice nurses, their primary focus and phenomena of concern are very different from each other. Whereas nurse practitioners are primarily responsible for direct patient care management, clinical nurse specialists are primarily responsible for ensuring the quality of nursing care for a population of patients.

Once the nurse dimensions of the Synergy Model are incorporated into job documents, the Synergy Model becomes the basis for hiring a new employee, for peer review, and for managerial evaluation. Yearly evaluation of nursing competence along the eight continuums of practice allows a more comprehensive assessment of an individual nurse's strengths and weaknesses. Depending upon the patient population, it is conceivable that certain aspects of practice would develop (or not) according to the needs of the patient population and available mentoring; for example, a staff nurse may possess level II competencies in clinical judgment but level I competence in clinical inquiry. While essential to the practice of nursing, having the opportunity to specifically comment during a peer review on a colleague's caring practices, collaboration, and systems thinking can be new to the evaluation scheme, especially in how it relates to team functioning.

Summarizing the yearly evaluations of all staff on a unit can serve to drive the professional development activities of the unit beyond completion of mandatory yearly reviews, maintenance of core competencies, and in-services on new products. Given the emphasis on nursing retention, it's imperative that staff development departments re-envision themselves as *professional* development departments with the goal of supporting the lifelong career development of staff. While several undergraduate and graduate programs use the Synergy Model as a conceptual framework, staff members welcome knowledge and skill development that supports professional growth in the nurse competencies described by the Synergy Model—clinical inquiry, for example. Centralized staff development departments can easily provide evidence-based practice workshops. An example of a successful workshop might include: (1) identifying a focused clinical question; (2) efficiently tracking down the best evidence to answer it; (3) critically appraising that evidence; (4) applying valid, useful evidence in practice; and (5) evaluating performance. After completion of the didactic content, staff can then participate in program-based, staff nurse III/clinical nurse specialist-led journal clubs to refine their skills in article critique.

Models of Care Delivery

Nursing needs a singular professional model of care and multiple care delivery models to capitalize on nursing expertise. Such a model enables them to prospectively plan and coordinate systems that help patients and families achieve desired outcomes in an efficient, cost-effective manner. Core values within the professional model of care include the primacy of patients, excellence in family-centered care, interdependency of multidisciplinary teams, mentoring staff, and reciprocal nurse "knowing the patient" and patient "knowing the nurse."

Although pockets of excellence exist, some patients still experience discontinuous care and nurses, especially the most expert, do experience unnecessary frustration. We are challenged to balance the needs of patients around the clock with staff nurses who possess differing levels of expertise and work schedules. Simply stated, a nurse is not a nurse is not a nurse. While nurses differentiate themselves based upon their evolving expertise, systems do not capitalize on it by affording them varying levels of professional autonomy and accountability for patient care.

In reality, everyone benefits from a care delivery model that is individualized, appropriate, anticipatory, coordinated, able to be evaluated, and cost effective. Primary objectives include:

- Eliminating unnecessary variation in care,
- Preventing interruptions in care through optimal team functioning,
- Enhancing relationships with patients and families (involvement, satisfaction, competence, and coping), and
- Increasing multidisciplinary collaboration and collegiality.

Objectives specific for nursing include:

- Increasing staff accountability,
- Increasing nurse autonomy,
- Developing staff competence at all levels, and
- Increasing staff satisfaction.

Because patients' needs and their trajectory of illness are different, a singular model of care delivery within any institution will not succeed in meeting everyone's needs. Adopting several models of care delivery and applying them based upon the individual needs of patients and families may help. In the mid 1990s, the nursing staff within the medical-surgical intensive care unit (ICU) at Children's Hospital Boston practiced traditional primary nursing. Recognizing the increasing frustration of all team members, the unit-based practice council used the Synergy Model as a framework to describe their patient population.

Three patient groups were identified:

1. Short-stay patients (length of stay less than 24 hours),
2. Typical ICU patients (length of stay 3 days), and
3. Chronically critically ill ICU patients (length of stay >2 weeks).

The fundamental needs of the three patient groups were very different. On one end of the spectrum, the short-stay patients were usually stable but vulnerable—they required a high level of nursing vigilance for early detection of any change in status; they experienced numerous transitions (admission, transfer, transport to diagnostic tests); and most families were very distressed and in need of almost continuous education and support. On the other end of the spectrum, the chronically critically ill patients were extremely complex, vulnerable, less resilient, and sometimes very unpredictable. In addition to daily updates, weekly multidisciplinary team meetings provided families with an opportunity to exchange information.

Two complementary models of care delivery, driven by patient and family needs, were designed for the unit: *team management* and *outcomes management*. Common features of each model included a "nurse attending" and up to five team members. In collaboration with the medical team, the nurse attending is accountable for the ongoing development, implementation, and evaluation of the nursing plan of care toward the delineated outcomes. The nurse attending assures that the plan of care is both individualized and prospectively developed so that all aspects of care occur in an anticipatory fashion to best meet the evolving needs of the patient and family. The nurse attending:

- Ensures the implementation of unit-based practice guidelines,
- Collaborates and coordinates the efforts of all the members of the multidisciplinary team in a manner that respects the unique contributions of each,
- Orchestrates team meetings at critical decision points,
- Keeps the family involved in making decisions and participating in the care process,
- Facilitates patient admission and discharge, and
- Mentors less experienced staff.

Patient populations targeted for team management included patients with a predictable trajectory of illness. Patient populations targeted for outcomes management were:

- Patients at high risk for a long, complicated, and/or erratic course of illness;
- Patients involved with multiple services (high variability in practice patterns); and
- Patients at high risk for complications. (See Table 1.1.)

Table 1.1. Linking Patient/Family Characteristics to a Model of Care Delivery.

Patient/Family Characteristic	Team Management	Outcomes Management
Physiological Stability	Stable to Unstable	Stable to Unstable
Complexity	Routine • Straightforward • Typical presentation • Simple dynamics	Complex • Ambiguous/vague, intricate • Atypical presentation • Intricate family dynamics
Vulnerability	Minimally vulnerable • Minimal risk	Vulnerable • Susceptible, unprotected, "at risk"
Predictability	Predictable • Usual and expected course • Generally follows trajectory	Unpredictable or predicted to have a complicated, protracted, and/or erratic course of illness • Uncommon, unusual, unexpected course
Resiliency	Resilient • Able to mount and maintain a response • Able to initiate some degree of compensation • Reserves	Minimally resilient • Unable to mount and maintain a response • Unable to initiate some degree of compensation • Limited reserves
Participation in Decision-Making and Care	Engaged/participating to minimal participation	Engaged/participating to minimal participation
Resource availability	Adequate to inadequate	Adequate to inadequate

Admitting and charge nurses work together to match individual patient needs to the care delivery model as soon as possible after ICU admission. All level I staff nurses can assume the team leader role. Outcomes managers are level II or III staff nurses who demonstrate proficient or expert clinical practice in all eight nurse dimensions of the Synergy Model. Specifically, they:

- Avoid the status quo,

- Envision the patient's needs and prospectively plan care,

- Demonstrate leadership,

- Take risks, are flexible, and bring teams together in the best interests of the patient,

- Partner with complex patients/families to define quality care/outcomes, and

- Interpret and analyze variance.

In addition to identifying nurses for the shift, the assignment board also contains information about the nurse's schedule. For example, working the 1st of 2 days, 2nd of 3 days, and so on. Charge nurses use this information about work schedule, level I and II/III status, and active teams to make assignments based on patients' needs for their *entire* ICU hospitalization. Nurses not involved in a team or working single shifts are assigned short-stay patients. While patient assignments determine team membership for team management, outcome managers play a more active role in building a patient's team of nurses based upon complementary skills and work schedules.

What is different is that patient needs are identified as soon as possible after admission, and then patients are matched to a care delivery model that makes sense for them and for the nurses. The unit's continuity of care index (number of different nurses providing care to the patient/number of nursing shifts experienced) and degree to which patients are receiving the appropriate model of care (team or outcomes) are monitored and reported to the unit's leadership council (Curley & Hickey, 2006).

Outcomes That Reflect the Nurse-Patient Relationship

Nursing's unique contribution to patients and their families—the contribution that encompasses all nurse competencies—is that nurses create safe passage for patients and their families (Curley, 1998). Safe passage, the outcome of a synergistic relationship, includes helping the patient and family move toward greater self-awareness and self-understanding, competence, and health, and through transitions and stressful events and/or a peaceful death.

Safe passage requires the nurse to know the patient/family and for the patient/family to know their nurse. Reciprocal (patient-nurse and nurse-patient) knowing requires organizational attention to a model of care delivery that provides continuity of care and opportunity for the nurse to spend time with the patient and family.

Outcomes related to limiting iatrogenic injury and complications to therapy acknowledge the potential hazards inherent in illness and the health-care environment. Nurses, through their clinical judgment and caring practices (vigilance), create healing environments that provide safe passage for vulnerable individuals. Nursing care rescues patients from anticipated complications and iatrogenic injury. A redefined "Failure to Rescue" (Silber, Williams, Krakauer, & Schwartz, 1992) outcome measure is an important outcome measure for the profession of nursing (Clarke & Aiken, 2003).

Consider using a safety metric that operationalizes patient safety to include how nurses keep the patient and the patient-care environment safe, such as nurse knowledge of the patient (see Box 1.2). This metric could address continuity of care, patient-nurse match, management plan-patient match, and perceived nursing workload. Unique to safety is a staff nurse interview that contains questions on nurse knowledge of the patient, nurse capacity to rescue the patient, and what nurses do to "rescue" patients from expected complications and/or untoward events.

Box 1.2. Safety Metric

"Safety" includes how nurses keep the patient and the patient-care environment safe—this includes nurse knowledge of the patient.

Part I

1. Continuity of care index: Number of nurses (a.) divided by the number of shifts (b.) the patient was hospitalized during the previous 7 days.
   a. Number of nurses: Please insert the total number of <u>assigned</u> nurses who cared for this patient during the patient's LOS (for up to 7 days). Include partial shifts as one full shift (for up to 7 days).

   b. Number of shifts: Please insert the total number of nursing shifts during the patient's LOS. Include partial shifts as one full shift.

OF THIS

    1) Number of nurses with <1 years of experience in the clinical area? (include per diem and travel nurses here).

    2) Number of nurses considered "clinical experts" <u>in the clinical area</u>?

2. Is there an identified nurse attending for this patient/family?

3. Patient needs, nursing expertise, and their match: In the past 24 hours only, please rate the following by checking the box corresponding to the number on the scales provided:

a. Compared with the other patients on the unit over the past 24 hours—THIS patient's acuity over the past 24 hours has been: Think about the patient's stability, complexity, vulnerability, predictability, resiliency, participation in decision-making and care, and resource availability.

Options:

-3	-2	-1	0	+1	+2	+3
Very Low			Neither high nor low		Very High	

b. Compared with the overall level of nursing expertise on the unit over the past 24 hours, the combined nursing expertise of the nurses who took care of THIS patient over the past 24 hours has been: Think about the collective nursing staff members' clinical judgment, clinical inquiry, caring practice, response to diversity, advocacy, facilitation of learning, collaboration, and systems thinking.

Options:

-3	-2	-1	0	+1	+2	+3
Very Low			Neither high nor low		Very High	

c. Over the past 24 hours, was this patient well matched to his/her assigned nurses' level of expertise?

Options: YES / NO

Part II - Staff Nurse Interview
(Conducted by a Level II/III Nurse)

Independent Assessment:

1. Does the patient's management plan reflect the patient's active problems? YES / NO

   Yes = complete so that a nurse who does not know the patient can take "good" care of the patient.

2. How many services are involved in this patient's care?

   1   2-3   4-6   >6

3. Given the patient's current state and the nurse's current assignment/workload, is this nurse able to be appropriately vigilant of this patient? YES / NO

Staff Nurse Interview:

1. Potential problem or problems jeopardizing this patient's recovery.

   Write in one problem:

   _____

   _____

   _____

   What symptoms would indicate that the patient had developed this problem? For example, ask "What symptoms are you looking for?" Write in up to 3 symptoms: (Does the interviewer agree with this? YES / NO)

   _____

   _____

   _____

   If these symptoms occurred, who (in addition to the charge nurse) would you notify?

   Name, Service, or Role (Does the interviewer agree with this? YES / NO)

   _____

   _____

   _____

   If necessary, do you have the necessary equipment on hand to deal with the problem? YES / NO / Not Applicable

2. Would you consider this patient at risk for a life-threatening problem?

   If yes—please specify one problem: (Does the interviewer agree with this? YES / NO)

   _____

If yes, who would you specifically notify if that problem occurred?

Name, Service, or Role (Does the interviewer agree with this?
YES / NO)

_____

If that individual didn't answer, how long would you wait before
going up the chain of command? ___ Minutes

If you disagreed with the resident's recommendations or
interventions, who specifically would you notify?

Name, Service, or Role (Does the interviewer agree with this?
YES / NO)

_____

Safe passage mandates preventive care—the prevention of iatrogenic injury, infection, and hazards of immobility, for example. Florence Nightingale (1890) noted that "*the purpose of nursing is to place the patient in the best position for nature to act upon him.*" The Critical Care and Cardiovascular Nursing Program at Children's Hospital Boston created "Nightingale Metrics" in each of its critical care and cardiovascular clinical areas (Curley & Hickey, 2006). The indicators were selected by staff nurses and include evidence-based independent and interdependent nursing activities that are required by their unique patient populations to put the patient in the best position for health and healing. Examples from the medical-surgical ICU include:

- Comfort assessment and management,
- Assessment and initiation of a nutrition plan,
- Patient positioning to prevent ventilator associated pneumonia and pressure ulcers,
- Deep vein thrombosis prophylaxis,
- Stress ulcer prophylaxis, and
- Discussion on rounds of the results of an extubation readiness testing and chemical paralysis honeymoon (when appropriate).

Linking the Nightingale Metrics with unit-based clinical outcome data will help make nursing visible within complex organizations.

Finally, the patient's and family's perception of being well cared for can be defined using the Synergy Model as a conceptual framework. Encompassing a wider construct than patient/family report of satisfaction, the patient's perception of being well cared for has not been operationally defined nor associated with any current measure. Yet, the fundamental premise of the Synergy Model is that patients drive nursing care. When patient characteristics and nurse competencies match and synergize, optimal patient outcomes may result. It makes sense that *when care is derived from what patients need*, it will be felt by them and contribute to their perception of being well cared for.

Curley and Hayes (2003) used focus group methodology to explore parents' perceptions of being cared for well. Each of the eight nurse dimensions of the Synergy Model were present in parent responses to the opening question: "What does it mean to you when you say that you and/or your child are cared for well by nurses?" Two of the eight dimensions of nursing practice were prominent; specifically, clinical judgment and caring practices were foundational to parent perceptions of being cared for well. When either dimension was lacking, parents did not experience being cared for well. Both clinical judgment and caring practices included concepts of vigilance. Clinical judgment also included knowing the specifics of a child's case and expected trajectory of illness. Caring practices included several humanistic concepts including being known, being respected as individuals, and being acknowledged as collaborators in their child's care. Feelings of trust, safety, and unburdening of the personal load of parent-to-a-sick-child are outcomes linked to the parent perceptions of being cared for well. Overall, parents clearly articulated a desired role for nurses and for themselves. As one parent noted: "The nurse is the connection. You start seeing the same ones over again. It's comforting to feel comfortable. You're comfortable with their experience, their level of care, and most importantly, their concern."

Sensitive measures that capture nursing and nurse-sensitive patient and family outcomes are essential for quality monitoring of nursing care and patient and family perceptions of care. The Synergy Model offers potential in advancing the measurement of nursing forward just beyond nurse-patient ratios or a dichotomous "primary nursing present" variable. Validating the dimensions of nursing practice that move patients toward specified outcomes in a measurable way will mean something to the patient, profession, employer, and society at large.

The Synergy Model in Context

Numerous mediating factors impact nurse-sensitive outcomes. First, optimal patient outcomes require both the unique and collective contributions of the patient and family, the nurse, the entire multidisciplinary team, and the health-care system. The health-care system in which this model will flourish is one that values and respects the contribution of nurses. These qualities are inherent in the core values of the Magnet Recognition Program—specifically, nursing empowerment, pride, mentoring, nurturing, respect, integrity, and teamwork (ANCC, 2004; Kramer & Schmalenberg, 1988; McClure & Hinshaw, 2002). The program objectives of Magnet designation include:

- Recognizing nursing services that use the *Scope and Standards for Nurse Administrators* (ANA, 2004b) to build programs of nursing excellence for the delivery of nursing care to patients,
- Promoting quality in a milieu that supports professional nursing practice,
- Providing a vehicle for the dissemination of successful nursing practices and strategies among health-care organizations using the services of registered professional nurses, and
- Promoting positive patient outcomes.

This truly is an exciting time for nursing. Health-care systems are focusing on best practice and on nursing recruitment and retention. Nursing's voice is universally clear on what stellar nursing care is. We now have the evidence to show that better patient and system outcomes result. Making nursing visible in today's health-care milieu demands that we have a clear sense of what nursing does, our relationship with patients and families, and our effect on patient outcomes. The Synergy Model gives voice to what patients collectively need and to what nurses collectively can do for humankind.

The AACN Synergy Model for Patient Care Revisited

Chapter 2

Martha A.Q. Curley, RN, PhD, FAAN

Originally published in 1998, the AACN Synergy Model for Patient Care™ describes patient-nurse relationships that are based on the needs of patients and their families (Curley, 1998). The fundamental premise of the Synergy Model is that patient characteristics drive nurse competencies. When patient characteristics and nurse competencies are in synergy, optimal patient outcomes are more apt to occur (see Figure 2.1).

Within this model, the patient and family are—or are assisted to become—active participants in the patient-family-nurse interaction. The interaction is synergistic. Specifically, it is reciprocating and coconstituting. The evolving relationship is characterized by responsive interdependence, intersubjectivity, shared commonality, and equity. The nurse comes to "know" the patient and family, and the patient and family come to "know" the nurse. When the relationship is in synchrony, when it is synergistic, optimal patient outcomes are more apt to occur.

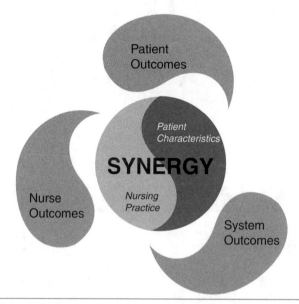

Figure 2.1.   The Synergy Model delineates three levels of outcomes:
patient outcomes, nurse outcomes, and system outcomes.
Used with permission. (Curley, 1998).

Patient Characteristics of Concern to Nursing

Each patient and family is unique, with varying capacities for health and vulnerability.
Individuals possess a singular genetic and biological make-up that establishes capacity
for health. Each individual practices varying degrees of healthy behaviors—for example,
healthy diets, exercise, and stress reduction. All individuals live in communities with different economic structures, government, social organization, and community perceptions.
All exist within a macro social structure consisting of societal infrastructure, physical
environment, cultural characteristics, and population perceptions (Tarlov, 1992). All these
factors place the patient in context of an individual within a unique environment and cir-
cumstance that impact the nursing care required of the particular patient and family.

Assumptions of the Synergy Model include:

1. The whole person is considered—body, mind, and spirit.

2. The context in which the nurse-patient interaction occurs impacts each dimension.
   Consideration is given to the patient/family/community biological, psychological,
   social, and spiritual dynamics, as well as the patient/family/community developmental stage.

3. The dimensions are not independent and cannot be considered in isolation. All are considered collectively to ascertain a quantifiable profile of the patient. This is also true of the nurse dimensions.

4. The goal of nursing is to restore the patient to an optimal level of wellness as defined by the patient and family. Death can be an acceptable outcome in which the goal of nursing care is to move the patient toward a peaceful death.

The Synergy Model describes a cluster of personal characteristics that each person brings to a health-care situation.

These eight characteristics span a continuum of health to illness and include:

1. Stability
2. Complexity
3. Vulnerability
4. Predictability
5. Resiliency
6. Participation in decision-making
7. Participation in care
8. Resource availability

Stability is the ability to maintain a steady state. Stability can be used to describe any vacillating phenomena that impact nursing care—physiological stability, psychological stability, emotional stability, and family or social stability.

Complexity is defined as the intricate entanglement of two or more systems. This characteristic includes multiple systems and/or therapies—body systems, family and social systems, and/or therapeutic interventions.

Vulnerability is a susceptibility to stressors that may adversely affect patient outcomes. Patient vulnerability considers the patient's risk for adverse outcomes. For example, individuals may present with comorbid conditions that place them at high risk for associated adverse outcomes (smoking and heart disease), and/or patients receiving certain therapies may be at risk for associated complications (chemotherapy and sepsis). Anticipatory assessment and management of associated risks or comorbid conditions impact the patient's nursing care and recovery.

Predictability is the characteristic that allows one to expect a certain trajectory of illness. While most patients have a predictable course of illness, some individuals do not respond in the typical fashion. When predictable, the patient's care can be managed using traditional practice guidelines; when unpredictable, practice guidelines are not helpful. Also, when the patient or the patient's diagnosis is unknown, one cannot anticipate his or her response to interventions or predict the trajectory of illness.

Resiliency is the capacity to return to a restorative level of functioning using compensatory and coping mechanisms. Some patients easily return to a stable state, while others do not. How a nurse approaches and plans interventions that may challenge the patient's stability is based upon the individual's capacity to restore homeostasis.

Participation in decision making describes the extent to which the patient or family engages in decision-making. The patient's and family's capacity, desire, and level of decision-making in daily management and overall treatment vary dramatically within the care environment. At different points during the illness, the nurse stands in for—or beside— a patient and family to support them though a decision that will impact their care and management.

Participation in care describes the extent to which the patient and family participate in care activities. Again, the patient's and family's capacity, desire, and level of participation in care vary dramatically within the care environment. At different points during the patient's illness, the nurse either provides or helps the patient and family give care.

Resource availability is the extent of resources the patient, family, or community brings to the care situation. Resources include personal, physiological, social, technical, and financial. The extent of available resources impacts the level of support nurses need to provide for patients and their families.

Patients and families vacillate along these eight continuums over time. For example, consider the case of a 30-year-old mother of two, recently divorced and relocated, with newly diagnosed uterine cancer undergoing chemotherapy. Her personal eight characteristics appear along the following continuum:

1. Stability can range from stable to unstable;
2. Complexity can range from simple to complex;
3. Vulnerability can range from minimally vulnerable to vulnerable;
4. Predictability can range from predictable to unpredictable;
5. Resiliency can range from resilient to less resilient;
6. Participation in decision making can range from engaged to minimally engaged;
7. Participation in care can range from participation to minimal participation; and
8. Resource availability can range from availability to low availability of resources.

Describing the patient's shifting points along these eight continuums paints a different picture of the patient and how a nurse would approach and care for the patient.

The Synergy Model lens is widened to consider the practice of advanced practice nurses or those in management positions. From the perspective of the clinical nurse specialist (CNS), nurse manager, clinical director, or vice president of nursing, the eight patient dimensions can be reconsidered and applied to the (a) nursing staff, (b) patient populations, and (c) systems that constitute the phenomena of concern for these nurses. For example, the stability, complexity, vulnerability, predictability, and resiliency of a particular program's nursing staff can be considered along with the extent to which the nursing staff typically participates in unit decision-making and care issues, and the resources available to the nursing staff. The patient population's stability, complexity, vulnerability, predictability, and resiliency can be considered along with the extent to which the population typically participates in decision-making and care, and the resources that are typically available to the population. Finally, the hospital system's stability, complexity, vulnerability, predictability, and resiliency can be considered along with the extent to which the system typically participates in decision-making and issues related to care, and the system resources that are typically available.

Nurse Competencies of Concern to Patients and Their Families

Nursing competencies, derived from the needs of patients, are also described in terms of essential continuums. The Synergy Model describes eight dimensions of nursing practice that span the continuum from competent to expert. These include: clinical judgment, clinical inquiry, caring practices, response to diversity, advocacy/moral agency, facilitation of learning, collaboration, and systems thinking. These competencies reflect a dynamic integration of knowledge, skills, experience, and attitudes needed to meet patient needs and optimize patient outcomes.

Clinical judgment is the ability of nurses to use their clinical knowledge to affect patient outcome. It is defined as clinical reasoning, which includes clinical decision-making, critical thinking, and a global grasp of the situation, coupled with nursing skills acquired through a process of integrating formal and experiential knowledge. Patricia Benner's *From Novice to Expert* (1984) has enriched how the nursing profession has come to understand clinical knowledge development. Clinical wisdom is not solely dependent on years of experience, but on experience gained from years of learning and applying knowledge gained to each successive patient.

Clinical inquiry involves resolving clinical problems that occur at the bedside and in the care environment. It is an ongoing process of questioning and evaluating practice, providing informed practice, and creating practice changes or innovation through research utilization and experiential learning. It is a matter of asking good questions, delving into the literature to answer those questions, and bringing the best evidence to the bedside. Whereas the competent nurse begins to question practice and compares and contrasts possible alternatives, the expert nurse is able to build a case for a change in practice based on data. Florence Nightingale was a pioneer in clinical inquiry. She identified clinical problems, collected data to first understand then build a case for change, and then redesigned models of care delivery that dramatically improved patient outcomes. Clinical inquiry is all about seeing, questioning, finding the evidence, and making practice changes.

Caring practices make our clinical judgment visible. These practices include a constellation of nursing activities that are responsive to the uniqueness of the patient and family and that create a compassionate and therapeutic environment with the aim of promoting comfort and preventing suffering. Caring practices, such as presence and vigilance, create a safe environment for patients to be sick in. Caring practices, extended to all members of the care team, create a therapeutic milieu. Family members feel cared for when they believe the nurse's vigilance matches the patient's need. Nurses, in sync with their patients, know when to be present, when to provide quiet space, and when to use humor in the patient-nurse relationship. Caring practices include not only what nurses do but how they do it. The primary fear of patients and their families is that the patient is going to experience unrelenting pain or that he or she will suffer. Pain assessment and management are fundamental caring activities. Caring practices also help make the worst thing a patient or family can possibly experience, the death of a loved one, a little more tolerable. Nurses are engaged during difficult situations, and they help the patient and families understand, approach, and manage these tough situations.

All patients are unique, with different values and beliefs that nurses learn so they can know what is important to the patient and his or her family. *Response to diversity* involves the sensitivity to recognize, appreciate, and incorporate differences in the provision of care. Differences may include, but are not limited to, individuality, culture, spiritual beliefs, gender, race, ethnicity, family configuration, lifestyle, socioeconomic status, age, values, and alternative medicine, involving patients/families and members of the health-care team. Nurses help families identify what is important and support them through difficult decisions. Whereas competent nurses inquire about differences and consider their impact on care, expert nurses tailor the environment to meet the diverse needs and strengths of the patient and family.

Advocacy/moral agency involves working on another's behalf, representing the concerns of the patient/family/community, and serving as a moral agent in identifying and helping to resolve ethical and clinical concerns within the clinical setting. Because of nursing's unique relationship with patients and families, nurses often are the voice for patients who cannot speak for themselves. Whereas competent nurses represent patients and their families when they cannot represent themselves, expert nurses carry on the moral tradition of nursing and serve as the patient's and family's moral agent: the person who takes a stand and gives voice to patient and family concerns.

Facilitation of learning refers to nurses' competency in facilitating patient, family, and staff learning. This includes supporting a learning environment characterized by safe discourse, mentoring, and team development. Teaching, along with patient and family learning, is embedded in care. From our first interaction, where we orient patients and family to the care environment, to our last interaction, where we finalize instructions for home self-care, nurses constantly teach. We also assume major responsibility for coaching and mentoring the next generation of nurses and members of the multidisciplinary team in the context-dependent aspects of care.

Collaboration includes working with others (patient, family, health-care providers, colleagues, community) in a way that promotes and encourages each person's contributions. Collaboration involves intradisciplinary and interdisciplinary work with colleagues and ability to negotiate and resolve conflict. The nurse is the one person who best knows the care environment and can pull a team of caregivers together for the best interest of the patient and family.

Systems thinking includes appreciating the care environment from a perspective that recognizes the interrelationships that exist within and across health-care settings. Making complex systems safe for patients is a skill. Whereas competent nurses operate on a micro level (unit and shift focus) and are just beginning to develop system savvy and strategies to facilitate change, expert nurses operate on a macro level (program and episode of illness focus), possess system savvy, and easily apply a variety of strategies to facilitate change within complex systems.

While competence in all dimensions is essential, nurses within subspecialties develop expertise within each dimension based on the typical needs of their patient population. For example, if the gestalt of the patient is stable but vulnerable, unpredictable, and minimally resilient, the primary nurse competencies would include at least a proficient level of clinical judgment and caring practices. If the gestalt of a patient is vulnerable, with minimal engagement in decision-making and care and inadequate resources, the primary competencies of the nurse would include at least a proficient level of advocacy, collaboration, and systems thinking. Competent to expert practice describes the "how" of nursing practice, while the Synergy Model describes the "what" of nursing practice.

The Synergy lens again widens to consider the practice of the clinical nurse specialist, nurse manager, clinical director, or vice president of nursing. The eight nurse dimensions are the same but reconsidered and applied to reflect individual responsibility to (a) nursing staff, (b) patient populations, and (c) systems that constitute the phenomena of concern.

Optimal Patient Outcomes

According to the Synergy Model, when patient characteristics and nurse competencies synergize, optimal patient outcomes result. Being kept in a primary position and having optimal outcomes are what patients themselves (or the people of significance to the patient) define as important. Three levels of outcomes are described: patient-level, unit-level, and system-level (see Table 2.1).

Table 2.1. Potential Outcomes of Patient/Family/Nurse Synergy

Patient and Family-Level Outcomes

- Symptom and disease management

  - Example: Improved pain, nausea, or dyspnea management
  - Example: Improved diabetes or asthma management

- Resolution of ethical problems

  - Example: Improved end-of-life decision-making

- Achievement of appropriate self-care

  - Example: Patient and family learning, patient and family competence in self-management, fewer delays in hospital discharge, and fewer patient readmissions in 30 days

- Demonstration of health-promoting behaviors

  - Example: Achievement of mutually acceptable goals; smoking cessation

- Health-related quality of life

  - Example: Improved functional health

- Rescue phenomena (Silber et al., 1992)

  - Example: Decreased impact of expected complications, early detection of unexpected complications, fewer hospital-acquired adverse events (urinary tract infections, central line infections, ventilator associated pneumonia, pressure ulcers, gastrointestinal bleeding, deep vein thrombosis, patient falls, errors), shorter acuity-adjusted length of stay (per DRG), improved risk-adjusted mortality (per DRG)

- Patient/family perception of being well cared for

  - Example: Improved patient/family trust in nursing staff, more patients and family can identify "their" nurse(s), improved patient/family satisfaction with their care experience.

Unit-Level Outcomes

- Shared accountability and authority for unit operations and performance

  - Example: More decisions made at the level of occurrence, more nurses actively participating in shared governance activities

- More experienced nurses catalyzing the advancement of less experienced nurses

  - Example: More coaching and mentoring, interest in advancing nursing education or in certification, creating unique educational opportunities to support practice (for example, sharing expertise with area schools of nursing)

System-Level Outcomes

- Nurse Satisfaction

  - Example: Improved nurse autonomy, perception of quality of care given, perception of adequate support services, time to do one's work, professional relationships, professional role enactment

- Staffing costs
  - Example: More nurse intent to stay, better retention of more experienced nurses, less turnover, decreased vacancy rates, less time to fill positions, shift to more hours worked per week, less absenteeism, reduced need for per diem staff
- Resource utilization and patient charges
  - Example: Less waste of supplies
- Multidisciplinary teamwork and satisfaction
  - Example: Improved measures of collaboration
- Cross-system innovation
  - Example: Improved system learning

Mitchell, Ferketich, & Jennings (on behalf of the American Academy of Nursing Expert Panel on Quality Health Care, 1998) described a Quality Health Outcomes Model that closely aligns the dynamic processes of patient care and outcomes. To best capture the unique contribution of nursing and care delivery models to patient/family well-being, Mitchell, Heinrich, Moritz, & Hinshaw (1997) proposed that outcome measures should integrate patients' experiences in health and illness. It was further proposed that outcome measures be operationalized in five categories: (1) symptom management, (2) achievement of appropriate self-care, (3) demonstration of health-promoting behaviors, (4) health-related quality of life, and (5) patient perception of being cared for well.

Encompassing a wider construct than patient/family report of satisfaction, the patient's perception of being cared for well has not been operationally defined or associated with any current measure. The Academy (Mitchell et al., 1997) recommended that there be work on a conceptual definition to broaden the concept beyond patient satisfaction and that considerable effort be put into achieving consensus for use of a standardized, clinically feasible instrument to promote comparisons and to determine sensitivity to change in organization factors. The patient's perception of being cared for well can be conceptually defined using the Synergy Model. The fundamental premise of the Synergy Model is that patients drive nursing care. When patient characteristics and nurse competencies match and synergize, optimal patient outcomes will likely result. It makes sense that when care is derived from what patients need, it will be felt by them and contribute to their perception of being cared for well.

Outcomes related to limiting iatrogenic injury and complications to therapy acknowledge the potential hazards inherent in illness and the health-care environment. Again, nurses, through their clinical judgment and caring practices (vigilance) create healing environments that provide safe passage for vulnerable individuals. Safe passage mandates preventive care, for example, the prevention of iatrogenic injury, infection, and hazards of immobility (e.g., pressure ulcers). Nursing care rescues patients from anticipated complications and iatrogenic injury. A redefined "Failure to Rescue" (Silber et al., 1992) outcome measure is an important outcome measure for the profession of nursing (Clarke & Aiken, 2003).

Nursing's unique contribution to patients and their families, the one that encompasses all nurse competencies, is that nurses create safe passage for patients and their families (Curley, 1998). Safe passage, the outcome of a synergistic relationship, includes helping the patient and family move toward greater self-awareness and self-understanding, competence, and health through transitions and stressful events, and/or a peaceful death.

Safe passage requires the nurse to know the patient and his or her family and the patient to know his or her nurse. Knowing the patient is a caring practice that includes knowing the patient and family as individuals and having an in-depth knowledge of their typical response (Tanner et al., 1993). Knowing the patient refers to how the nurse understands the patient, grasps the meaning of the situation for the patient, and recognizes the need for a particular intervention. Knowing the patient requires clinical judgment and creates possibility for advocacy that limits the patient vulnerability and prevents iatrogenic injury. Reciprocal (patient-nurse and nurse-patient) knowing requires organizational attention to a model of care delivery that provides continuity of care and opportunity for the nurse to spend time with the patient and family.

Numerous mediating factors impact patient-nurse-system outcomes. First, optimal outcomes require both the unique and collective contributions of the patient and family, the nurse, and the entire multidisciplinary team. The health-care system directly impacts the nurse-patient relationship, and thus will directly influence the Synergy Model outcomes.

In conclusion, this chapter provides an update on the Synergy Model. Acknowledging the primacy of nursing based upon the needs of patients and their families has a long tradition in nursing. The fundamental premise of the Synergy Model is that patient characteristics drive nurse competencies. When patient characteristics and nurse competencies are in synergy, optimal patient outcomes are more apt to occur.

Using the Synergy Model to Describe Nursing Work and Progressive Levels of Practice

Anne Micheli, RN, MSN
Martha A.Q. Curley, RN, PhD, FAAN

Children's Hospital Boston is a 340-bed center for pediatric health care that offers a complete range of services for pediatric patients from 15 weeks' gestation through 21 years of age. With more than 30 clinical departments and 150 subspecialty programs, nurses at Children's Hospital Boston believe in the primacy of patients and families (the individual needs of patients and families drive nursing care) and that excellence in care is provided through meaningful therapeutic relationships with patients and their families. The advancement of nursing practice is one of the cornerstones of the philosophy of nursing at the hospital.

Children's Hospital Boston has had a formal Professional Advancement Program for more than 20 years (Balasco & Black, 1988). The goal of the program is to recognize and reward nurses for advancing levels of practice and to promote a lifelong career approach to nursing by supporting professional advancement based on clinical expertise, individual accomplishment, and contribution to patient care and unit activities.

Program Genesis

The program was developed in 1985 by the newly formed Professional Advancement Committee soon after publication of Patricia Benner's (1984) book, *From Novice to Expert*. Dr. Benner categorized five incremental levels of clinical proficiency found in nursing practice: novice, advanced beginner, competent, proficient, and expert. The levels reflect a change in two aspects of skilled performance. One is a movement from reliance on abstract principles to the use of past, concrete experience. The other is a change in the perception and understanding of a situation so that the situation is seen less as a compilation of equally relevant bits and more as a complete whole in which certain parts are relevant.

Using Dr. Benner's work as a foundation, Children's Hospital Boston defined three levels of practice: level I competent, level II proficient, and level III expert. Behavioral criteria describing these three levels of practice were defined by the Professional Advancement Committee with approval of the Nursing Leadership Council and were incorporated into the staff nurse I, II, and III job documents. At that time the behavioral criteria were written in four domains: clinical practice, clinical leadership, professional growth, and quality improvement with an emphasis on the nurse rather than on the patient. Upon completion, we invited Dr. Benner to review our program; she enthusiastically endorsed our advancement process and criteria, noting that it truly embodied her work.

Staff Nurse Levels

Staff Nurse I represents a competent level of professional practice. Nurses in this position identify opportunities for continued professional development that correspond with their personal career goals. Nurses can choose to remain at this level throughout their career or seek advancement to staff nurse II.

Staff Nurse II represents a proficient level of practice characterized by specialized clinical knowledge and skill. Staff nurse II is a recognized role model, clinical resource, and leader who demonstrates commitment to achieving unit goals.

Staff Nurse III represents an expert level of practice characterized by the ability to direct, support, and influence nursing practice within the institution. The staff nurse III takes an active part in the achievement of program goals.

The advancement process from level I to level II is unit based. Interest in advancement is first discussed during the staff nurse's peer review and annual performance evaluation. Peer and manager support is affirmed before the candidate's formal application. The candidate compiles a portfolio. The portfolio includes a letter of intent to apply for promotion, a statement of practice (narrative statement that reflects the candidate's nursing philosophy and provides evidence of level II practice), one clinical exemplar, and evidence of peer support. The nurse manager reviews the candidate's portfolio for evidence of level II behaviors, and if present, promotes the candidate. The staff nurse II receives a salary differential upon promotion.

The advancement process from level II to level III is both unit and department based. Again, peer and manager support is affirmed before the candidate's formal application. The candidate creates a portfolio that includes a letter of intent, current curriculum vitae, statement of practice, two clinical exemplars, letters of support for promotion, and appendices illustrating his or her best practices/work. Copies of the portfolios are distributed to the members of the board of review 10 days before the review. The staff nurse III also receives a salary differential upon promotion.

The board of review is composed of the chair/facilitator and eight level III staff nurses appointed by the vice president of patient care services. Members of the board represent the diversity of practice at Children's Hospital Boston. As the number of candidates increased over the years, the board of review meeting times increased from quarterly to monthly. The meeting starts in closed session, with a review of the candidate's materials. In open session the candidate and his or her manager provide statements highlighting the candidate's practice, specifically noting how the candidate meets level III criteria. The general mood of the board of review is celebratory, as it truly functions to help individuals recognize and reward their personal achievement. Members develop a high level of expertise in this process over time and acquire skills in putting the candidate at ease and eliciting discussion that best reveals the candidate's level of practice and accomplishment. Board membership is rotated, and more experienced members mentor new members.

Synergizing the Professional Advancement Program

The Professional Advancement Program withstood the test of time because it resonated with the mission and vision of the organization. However, the behavioral criteria needed to be broadened to better reflect the primacy of patients, contemporary nursing practice within a complex organization, interdisciplinary work and the evolving focus on patient and family outcomes. The importance of the staff nurse role in recruiting, retaining, teaching, and mentoring colleagues also needed to be considered. The AACN Synergy Model for Patient Care™ added the dimensions of caring practices, response to diversity, advocacy/moral agency, facilitation of learning, collaboration, and systems thinking to our core competencies of clinical judgment and clinical inquiry.

In January 2000, the Professional Advancement Committee began work on revising the three staff nurse job documents based on the Synergy Model. AACN descriptors were used as a foundation but expanded to reflect pediatric nursing practice and the continuum of practice from ambulatory to critical care nursing. Criteria were written to reflect a non-linear, nonincremental advancement in practice with the assumption that the staff nurses demonstrate behaviors at the previous level before advancement.

Members of the Professional Advancement Committee developed the new criteria over several months. Focused input was sought from special-interest groups; for example, the Ethics Committee for the advocacy/moral agency dimension, the Education Council for facilitation of learning dimension, and the Pain Committee and Family Center for the caring practices dimension.

Once we had a working document that included three levels for all eight dimensions, the Professional Advancement Committee sponsored four town meetings. These open forums not only provided information about the anticipated change in the job documents and in the Synergy Model, but provided the opportunity for members of the Professional Advancement Committee to receive feedback on the evolving content of each new dimension. The revised job documents were presented to the Staff Nurse Council for review and comment.

Drafts of the working job document were formally reviewed by the nurse directors, nurse managers, and staff nurses responsible for yearly evaluations. Reviewers were asked to evaluate each criteria/descriptor for 1) the extent to which that descriptor accurately described the dimension (5 point scale), 2) the extent to which that descriptor accurately described the level of practice within that dimension at Children's Hospital Boston (5 point scale), and 3) the importance of that descriptor in that dimension (rank order). The Professional Advancement Committee reviewed the results and modified the working job documents.

The working job documents were then presented at a joint Leadership Staff Nurse Council retreat conducted by members of the Committee. The purpose of this meeting was to discuss, approve, and finalize each document (see Table 3.1, staff nurse I, II, and III criteria).

The Professional Advancement Program then hosted eight 2-hour interrater reliability sessions for each dimension of the job documents. The goal of these sessions was to reach agreement in citing examples of practice that illustrate each behavior listed in the staff nurse I, II, and III job documents. When the sessions were completed, we had examples of performance expectations that allowed nurses to be promoted across the system in an equitable fashion.

Initially we simply inserted the new job content into our standard evaluation tool, but during the implementation phase, it became immediately clear that the new job document was lengthy and cumbersome to complete, as it retained some nonevaluatory information and now had eight dimensions versus four domains. The evaluation tool was then reformatted and condensed to improve its usability.

The process for advancement was slightly redefined to incorporate Synergy Model language. The process for advancement to level II remains unit based and the process for advancement to level III remains departmental with the board of review. The level II and III portfolios should demonstrate that the candidate meets the criteria for each dimension of the Synergy Model. The level III candidate's meeting with board members further substantiates the candidate's level of practice.

The Synergy Model for evaluation and advancement has placed the emphasis on clinical practice and is patient-nurse focused. The criteria are clearly written and are relevant in every clinical area of practice in Children's Hospital Boston. The job document can be used as a peer review tool, as well as the evaluation tool for the nurse manager.

The board of review members for advancement to level III have found that the Synergy Model has made the portfolio and candidate review much easier, because the required elements of practice for advancement in each dimension can be quickly identified. Portfolios better reflect the commitment to excellence and passion for patient care and clinical expertise. The dimensions also allow for the description of how a nurse positively affects patient care by mentoring and collaborating with colleagues. Candidates who use the Synergy Model for the statement of practice and clinical exemplars can clearly describe how they meet the criteria.

Upon completion of the staff nurse I, II, and III job documents, new documents were created for the nurse manager (see Table 3.2), advanced practice nurse (see Table 3.3), and nursing research director roles (see Table 3.4). They were modeled after the staff nurse documents, and each was created by the individuals serving in those roles. Using one framework for all departmental job documents allows one to compare the fundamental similarities and differences describing the work of nursing within an organization.

Table 3.1.   Staff Nurse I, II, and III

From the Professional Advancement Committee, Children's Hospital Boston, 2007. Used with permission.

Clinical Judgment

STAFF NURSE I	STAFF NURSE II	STAFF NURSE III
Conducts accurate clinical assessments. Identifies and prioritizes patient/family needs. Develops, implements, and evaluates the nursing plan of care. Modifies plan to meet established clinical outcomes. Follows algorithms, decision trees, and protocols. Integrates formal knowledge with clinical events to make decisions. Seeks validation for own clinical decisions. Integrates input from other clinicians for decision-making. Delegates tasks/care to appropriate staff and ensures timely follow-up.	Easily applies, modifies, and reinforces clinical guidelines to meet individual patient/family needs. Collects and interprets complex patient data. Focuses on key elements of situation while sorting out extraneous details. Exercises clinical judgment based on an immediate grasp of the whole picture for program-specific patient populations. Anticipates and recognizes subtle cues, patterns, and trends that may predict the direction of illness. Serves as a coach in evaluating and validating colleagues' clinical judgment. Comfortable seeking multidisciplinary consultation.	Rapidly synthesizes and interprets multiple, sometimes conflicting, sources of data. Makes judgments based on an immediate grasp of the whole picture. Uses formal and experiential knowledge to anticipate problems for complex patient populations within and beyond program in area of expertise. Uses innovative strategies to achieve clinical outcomes. Assumes a leadership role in assisting patient and family teamwork toward short- and long-term goals. Comfortable relying on intuitive knowledge. Recognizes and plans for evolving patterns in patient populations.

Clinical Inquiry

STAFF NURSE I	STAFF NURSE II	STAFF NURSE III
Asks questions to clarify understanding on current practice. Selects and follows clinical practice guidelines, protocols, and algorithms. Supports the implementation of clinical changes and evidence-based practices. Participates in quality/performance improvement initiatives.	Continually questions current practice to meet patients' needs. Compares, contrasts, and evaluates possible alternatives. Identifies clinical questions. Seeks advice, resources, or information to improve patient care. Contributes to the development of hospital- and unit-based clinical practice guidelines.	Conveys advanced knowledge and skills needed to address problems arising in practice and improve patient care. (The domains of clinical judgment and clinical inquiry converge at the expert level; they are not separable). Uses an evidence-based process to evaluate current practices and make recommendations for best practices. Provides leadership in the development of clinical practice guidelines. Provides leadership in implementing best practices.

Caring Practices

STAFF NURSE I	STAFF NURSE II	STAFF NURSE III
Interacts with patients and families in a compassionate and humanistic manner, demonstrating empathy, sensitivity, and patience.	Consistently shows empathy, sensitivity, and insight and is able to intervene in difficult, stressful, or volatile situations.	Preserves, protects, and enhances the environment that supports caring.
Maintains a safe and caring environment for both patient and family.	Detects and responds to subtle patient and family changes.	Provides comforting practices that follow the patient and family lead.
Manages both emotional and physical pain and promotes comfort based on standards and protocols.	Tailors pain management and comfort measures to the individuality of patient and family.	Anticipates and plans for patient and family needs and potential problems as they transition along the health-care continuum. Works with staff to help patients and families to maintain their own optimal level of care.
Develops therapeutic relationships with patient and family and maintains appropriate boundaries.	Models therapeutic relationships with patient and family that facilitate mutual involvement in planning of care.	Orchestrates the process that enables the comfort of patients and families surrounding all possible outcomes.
Acknowledges that a patient's clinical outcome may be less than optimal.	Assists the patient, family, and staff in acknowledging that a clinical outcome may be less than optimal.	Creates an environment that fosters mutual respect and professional growth.
	Contributes to a nurturing environment that is supportive to/of colleagues.	

Response to Diversity

STAFF NURSE I	STAFF NURSE II	STAFF NURSE III
Recognizes unique differences of patient and family and incorporates them into an individualized plan of care.	Anticipates and integrates cultural differences into patient and family care.	Mentors colleagues in incorporating differences into the provision of care.
Delivers care in a nonjudgmental and nondiscriminatory manner.	Makes provisions and helps advocate for patient and family requests for incorporating alternative therapies into care.	Tailors health-care culture to meet the diverse needs and strengths of the patient and family.
Assesses patient and family level of understanding to provide effective communication.	Assists staff in recognizing and incorporating differences among team members into the plan of care and care environment.	Anticipates differences and beliefs within the team and negotiates consensus in the best interest of the patient and family.
Tailors nursing care to meet the age-specific and developmentally appropriate needs of patient and family.	Cognizant of one's own beliefs and values and recognizes their potential influence on nursing practice.	Promotes an environment that recognizes and supports the unique contributions of staff.

Advocacy/Moral Agency

STAFF NURSE I	STAFF NURSE II	STAFF NURSE III
Preserves and protects the confidentiality, autonomy, dignity, and rights of patient and family.	Acts as a resource in helping patients and families work toward resolution of ethical conflict.	Anticipates ethical choices and prepares patient and family as well as clinical team.
Completes assessments and formulates an individualized plan to accurately reflect patient and family values and goals, so they can be fully represented in care.	Initiates an ethics consult when appropriate.	Advocates from perspective of patient and family and works toward resolution of complex ethical conflicts.
Works on behalf of all patients and families. Seeks help to represent patients and families when they are unable to represent themselves.	Applies ethical principles in supporting the moral and legal rights of patients and families.	Consistently establishes professional relationships with patient and family that are characterized by mutual respect.
Raises ethical questions and concerns with clinical team. Seeks available resources to help formulate and understand ethical decisions.	Provides support to colleagues and families during moral conflict and compromise.	Advocates on behalf of a specific population of patients.
		Cultivates an environment that is supportive of colleagues' development in ethical reasoning.
		Participates in institutional organizational mechanisms for dealing with clinical ethical problems.

Facilitator of Learning

STAFF NURSE I	STAFF NURSE II	STAFF NURSE III
Integrates patient and family education throughout the delivery of care. Helps patients and families learn what they need to successfully transition within the health-care environment.	Recognizes and integrates unique ways of teaching that complement patient and family learning needs.	Modifies, develops, and evaluates program-based patient and family education.
Assesses and then documents the learning needs of patients and families. Collaborates with peers in establishing individualized teaching plans.	Coordinates and incorporates health-care providers' perspectives and plans into patient and family education.	Assists patients, families, and staff in complex, challenging situations in developing individualized education plans.
Provides patient and family with appropriate information to help them participate and/or make informed decisions about their health care and treatments, including health promotion and disease prevention.	Expands network of educational resources for patient and family within the hospital and community.	Monitors the learning needs of staff and provides educational opportunities and strategies to enhance knowledge and skills of colleagues.
	Serves as a resource in designing teaching plans for patients and families; provides guidance, instruction and support for peers.	Creates and seeks opportunities to coach and mentor and to be taught, coached, and mentored.

Facilitator of Learning (continued)

STAFF NURSE I	STAFF NURSE II	STAFF NURSE III
Uses available educational resources within the hospital and community for patients and families.	Evaluates effectiveness of educational plans for program-specific population groups.	Serves as a model for professional practice within a program and as a resource for the clinical specialty outside the program.
Validates and documents patient and family learning.	Actively seeks learning opportunities and establishes coaching and mentoring relationships.	Establishes outcome measures to systematically evaluate the effectiveness of family education programs.
Shares own knowledge with colleagues.		
Identifies personal goals and seeks opportunities to pursue professional growth.		

Collaboration

STAFF NURSE I	STAFF NURSE II	STAFF NURSE III
Functions as a team member and works collaboratively and interdependently.	Demonstrates initiative when working with team toward achievement of optimal patient, family, and staff outcomes.	Creates an environment that facilitates collaboration on multiple dimensions to improve quality of care to populations of patients and families.
Open and sensitive to all team members' unique contributions.	Models leadership behavior in an interdisciplinary manner that invites utilization by colleagues.	Coaches staff in making decisions that involve diverse disciplines to optimize outcomes.
Uses resources to develop and implement an integrated plan of care.	Effectively communicates and negotiates needed changes in a patient's plan of care.	Facilitates active involvement and complementary contributions of others in meetings and activities regarding patient care and practice issues.
Receptive to being taught, coached, and mentored.	Uses positive mechanisms that reflect insight into own behavior to work toward resolution of conflict.	Identifies and works toward resolution of conflict that affects performance, without making any party feel diminished.
Delegates to assistive and other personnel in a manner that optimizes patient care.		
Receptive to discussing issues that work toward resolution of conflict.		

Systems Thinking

STAFF NURSE I	STAFF NURSE II	STAFF NURSE III
Uses a familiar array of strategies and available clinical resources for problem-solving.	Integrates all aspects of patient care. Promotes continuity in care by effectively anticipating, planning, and managing patient transitions across the care continuum.	Develops, integrates, and applies a variety of problem-solving strategies that are driven by the needs and strengths of the patient, family, and program.
Assumes an active role in keeping informed about changes in hospital policy, procedure, and equipment.	Anticipates and initiates timely referral and follow-up to ensure needed services for patient and family transition.	Demonstrates a global and holistic perspective that expands from the care setting to the entire health-care system.
Recognizes that resources are limited and evaluates factors related to safety, effectiveness, and cost when two or more practice options would result in the same expected outcome.	Develops problem-solving strategies based on the unique needs and strengths of a particular patient and family. Negotiates to reach agreement.	Recognizes system failures and knows when and how to negotiate and navigate through the system on behalf of patients, families, and staff.
	Demonstrates leadership ability when responding to situations and efficiently uses existing resources. Uses untapped and alternative clinical resources as necessary.	Analyzes competing demands and provides leadership in system redesign to best meet the needs of patients, families, and staff.
	Helps develop, select, and/or evaluate new resources.	Analyzes current system and develops strategies to enhance resources.
	Creates opportunities to improve efficiency of operations and quality of services. Balances competing demands. Recognizes system failures and participates in problem resolution.	Develops innovative strategies to enhance communication throughout the health-care system.

Table 3.2.   Nurse Manager

From the Nurse Manager Council, Children's Hospital Boston, 2007. Used with permission.

CLINICAL JUDGMENT

1. Contributes to an environment that facilitates development of clinical expertise of staff by role modeling, teaching, and coaching/mentoring.
2. Uses knowledge and expertise to identify potential problems and/or resources for patients and families.
3. Ensures that all staff members maintain level of competency-based practice based upon patient population.

CLINICAL INQUIRY

1. Anticipates and identifies evidence-based opportunities for improvement that promote practice and change.
2. Develops and implements a performance-improvement program for area(s) of responsibility.
3. Enhances evidence-based practice; maintains knowledge and skills through professional growth.
4. Identifies, proposes, and conducts clinical research.
5. Manages or supervises unit/department personnel by evaluating work performance, providing guidance, and giving feedback based on outcome measures.

CARING PRACTICES

1. Assists in the coordination of patient care conferences with staff to help ensure best caring practices and outcomes for patients and families.
2. Participates in interdisciplinary rounds to address caring practices, patient and family needs, and discharge planning.
3. Fosters patient, family, and professional relationships that are reciprocal, synergistic, and characterized by mutual respect and professional growth.
4. Cultivates an environment that is supportive of staff's professional and personal growth.

RESPONSE TO DIVERSITY

1. Identifies issues arising from individual differences and develops awareness of these issues in nursing staff, medical staff, and other health-care providers.
2. Role models, teaches, and/or provides age-specific and developmentally appropriate patient care in accordance with established guidelines and scope of duty or practice for patients served in program.
3. Identifies and resolves conflicts between others that affect performance, without making any party feel diminished.

ADVOCACY/MORAL AGENCY

1. Advocates on behalf of the nursing staff to represent the concerns of patients, families, and staff.
2. Works in collaboration with multidisciplinary team to balance technology with values that emphasize quality of life, consumer choice, risk-benefit decisions, access, and integrity of human life.

3. Provides leadership in creating an ethical practice environment for professional practice and patient care based on optimum communication and coordination of care.

4. Supports proactive identification and addressing of ethical issues through a systematic process using institutional ethics committees as needed.

5. Promotes pediatric health care at local, state, national, and international levels.

FACILITATOR OF LEARNING

1. Modifies, develops, and evaluates program-based education programs for the patient and family.

2. Monitors the learning needs of staff and designs educational opportunities to enhance knowledge and skills of colleagues.

3. Serves as a mentor for professional practice.

4. Functions as an expert resource within and outside clinical specialty program.

5. Identifies avenues to pursue own professional growth.

COLLABORATION

1. Role models, teaches, and/or mentors professional leadership and accountability for nursing's role within the health-care team.

2. Designs, implements, and evaluates specified program of caregiving in collaboration with other programs.

3. Leads and participates in departmental and hospital programs, committees, and special projects to achieve desired outcomes.

SYSTEMS THINKING

1. Recognizes, responds, and provides follow-up for all issues, concerns, and suggestions on behalf of the patient population and staff.

2. Provides timely follow-up on critical incidents and sentinel events and provides leadership in system redesign to promote a culture of safety for patients, families, and staff.

3. Analyzes and prioritizes competing demands, taking effective action to redesign systems to best meet the needs of a patient population and staff.

4. Assumes accountability for daily operations at the unit level.

5. Allocates resources and coordinates services to optimize patient care and services.

6. Assists in developing and monitoring the operating and capital budget, resolves variances, implements strategies to improve efficiency and reduce costs.

7. Integrates knowledge of organizational mission, goals, and systems into staff and patient strategies, development, and implementation.

Table 3.3.   Advanced Practice Nurse

From the Nurse Practitioner and Clinical Nurse Specialist councils, Children's Hospital Boston, 2007.
Used with permission.

Nurse Practitioner	Clinical Nurse Specialist
Clinical Judgment:	
Synthesizes and interprets multiple sources of data, in collaboration with the health-care team.	Clinical reasoning is recognized at an expert level.
Makes accurate clinical diagnosis and formulates an individual treatment plan with expected outcome. Evaluates treatment, and revises treatment plan as necessary.	Anticipates, synthesizes, interprets, makes decisions, and evaluates responses based on complex and sometimes conflicting sources of data.
	Predicts the clinical course and takes the lead in developing preventive nursing interventions to improve clinical outcomes for complex patient situations.
Performs needed diagnostic and therapeutic procedures as indicated within scope of practice, and prescribes appropriate medications within scope of practice privileges. members	Assists all members of the health-care team in recognizing the patient's overall condition. Facilitates the clinical judgment of all of the health-care team.
Provides leadership in the development, implementation and evaluation of algorithms, decision trees, and practice protocols. Helps to develop the clinical judgment of other health-care team members.	Develops, implements, and/or evaluates research-based algorithms, decision trees, protocols, and pathways for patient populations.
	Serves as expert resource to all members of the multidisciplinary team regarding patient and program issues.
Clinical Inquiry:	
Uses research-based evidence and outcome data to formulate, evaluate, and/or revise treatment plans, policies, procedures, and standards of care.	
Assumes a leadership role in recommending, implementing, and evaluating evidence-based practice.	Integrates knowledge, research findings, and experience to enhance nursing clinical practice and to promote excellence in patient care.
Develops and conducts research/outcome studies to optimize patient care and cost-benefit ratios and evaluate patient care issues, problems, and products and technology.	Develops, monitors, and/or evaluates QI projects on a unit and hospital level using quality outcomes indicators.
	Mentors staff in critiquing literature to determine applicability to practice.
Role models, teaches, coaches, and/or mentors nursing staff regarding the use and evaluation of research findings.	Develops and/or participates in research/ outcome studies to evaluate patient care issues, products, and technology.

Nurse Practitioner	Clinical Nurse Specialist

Caring Practices:

Models therapeutic relationships with the patient and family that facilitate mutual involvement in planning care. Empowers patients and families to maintain their own optimal level of care.

Participates in establishing a caring environment for patients, families, and staff.

Assists the patient and family in acknowledging expected and actual outcomes.

Reduces barriers to patient and family wellness (i.e., place patient and family in an optimal environment to heal).

Contributes to the establishment of an environment that promotes caring and diminishes feelings of powerlessness/suffering.

Interprets and communicates complex patient and family needs to other caregivers.

Cares for the caregiver (e.g., conflict resolution, debriefing, and crises intervention). Preserves, protects, and enhances the environment that supports human dignity.

Cares for the caregivers (i.e., facilitates conflict resolution, conducts debriefing sessions and crisis intervention).

Facilitates colleagues' development of caring practices through role modeling, teaching, coaching, and mentoring.

Response to Diversity:

Integrates the unique concerns and value system of patient, family, nursing staff, and team into patient's plan of care.

Role models, teaches, coaches, and/or mentors acceptance of and responsiveness to unique care needs of patient and family.

Identifies evolving trends arising from individual differences and initiates development of an intervention to accommodate differences.

Tailors the delivery of care to meet the diverse needs and strengths of patient, family, staff, and system.

Advocacy/Moral Agency:

Creates an environment that supports the patient, family, and staff in representing themselves.

Assists the patient, family, and nursing staff in representing themselves.

Provides patients and families with appropriate information to help them participate and/or make informed decisions about health care and treatments, including health promotion and disease prevention.

Facilitates development of nurses' advocacy and moral agency through role modeling, teaching, coaching, and/or mentoring.

Recognizes the moral and legal rights of emancipated minors and adults and the emerging rights of mature minors, as well as parental rights.

Contributes to staff knowledge of ethical issues common to one's clinical area.

Anticipates ethical conflicts and prepares patient and family, as well as clinical team.

Contributes to an environment that promotes ethical decision-making and patient advocacy.

Supports colleagues and families during ethical conflict. Utilizes appropriate resources, e.g., Ethics Committee.

Cultivates an environment that is supportive of colleagues' development in moral agency and ethical reasoning.

Nurse Practitioner	Clinical Nurse Specialist

Facilitator of Learning:

Integrates patient and family education throughout the delivery of care. Incorporates disease and injury presentation, health promotion, and health maintenance issues in the treatment plan.	Assesses learning needs of staff and provides formal and informal educational opportunities to improve staff knowledge and enhance clinical performance. Collaborates in the development, implementation, and/or evaluation of unit-based and specialty-based competencies.
Synthesizes interdisciplinary care recommendations and educational plans into the patient and family education process.	Collaborates in the refinement of education programs for both patients and nurses based on program-specific goals.
	Facilitates nursing staffs' development of patient and family education and skills.
Assesses the learning needs of colleagues and designs educational opportunities to enhance knowledge and skills of colleagues.	Provides guidance for professional advancement to staff nurses.
Serves as a mentor for professional practice and as a resource for colleagues.	Coordinates formal and informal intra-disciplinary and interdisciplinary education to improve patient outcomes and quality of care.
Contributes to the knowledge base of the profession and specialty programs through publications, presentations, and participation in the work of professional organizations.	Establishes outcome measures to systematically evaluate the effectiveness of educational programs.
	Establishes an active professional involvement with the academic community (i.e., participating in collegiate programs, precepting students, and other related activities).
Critically evaluates one's own professional practice. Actively and regularly seeks experiences and learning opportunities that will advance one's own knowledge of interventions, therapeutics, and clinical skills. Verbalizes and documents advanced nursing practice in an articulate and comprehensive manner.	Contributes to and advances nursing knowledge through presentations, publications, and involvement in professional organizations.

Collaboration:

Collaborates with other caregivers and various disciplines as needed to comprehensively address patient and family health needs.	Role models, coaches, teaches, and mentors nursing staff to understand and use resources and expertise of others.
Models a professional relationship that invites utilization and collaboration with colleagues.	Mentors nurses in professional leadership and accountability for nursing practice.
Guides colleagues in making clinical and management decisions that involve and recruit diverse disciplines when appropriate to optimize patient outcomes.	Maintains collaborative relationships among teams to facilitate intradisciplinary and interdisciplinary practice.

Nurse Practitioner	Clinical Nurse Specialist

Collaboration (continued):

Works with community agencies (physicians, VNA, schools, Medicaid, etc.) to coordinate care. Initiates and facilitates active involvement with external agencies (e.g., industry, insurers, community groups) related to clinical practice area.

Leads multidisciplinary teams in developing programs focused on patient care, staff, and/or system issues.

Critically evaluates the professional practice of other health-care team members, providing constructive feedback as necessary.

Systems Thinking:

Integrates knowledge of organizational mission, goals, and systems into patient care.

Develops problem-solving strategies based on the unique needs and strengths of a particular patient and family.

Applies expert knowledge of the system and works with the entire team to optimize patient care delivery and patient safety.

Responds to situations with an efficient use of existing resources. Participates in the development of new cost-effective resources.

Role models, teaches, coaches, and/or mentors creative problem-solving and utilization of resources among staff.

Creates opportunities to improve the efficiency of operations and quality of services. Balances competing demands. Recognizes system failures and participates in problem-solving.

Develops innovative strategies to facilitate optimal patient transition through the health-care system (e.g., decrease LOS)

Anticipates possible consequences of systems change and develops proactive strategies to enhance implementation.

Assumes responsibility to build systems to improve patient care and patient care delivery.

Understands and completes all requirements for credentialing and privileging of advanced practice nurses within the Children's Hospital system.

Assumes proactive role in system redesign that supports a safe environment for staff, patients, and families.

Table 3.4. Nursing Research Director

From Children's Hospital Boston, 2007. Used with permission..

Clinical Judgment

1. Clinical reasoning is exemplary.
2. Evaluates phenomena based on complex and sometimes conflicting sources of data.
3. Advances the clinical judgment skills of the nursing staff within designated area of responsibility.
4. Assists in development and evaluation of research-based algorithms, decision trees, protocols, and pathways for patient populations.
5. Serves as the nursing science expert in designated area of responsibility.

Clinical Inquiry

1. Mentors staff in using the best available evidence when solving patient care problems and/or developing policies, procedures, protocols, and standards of care.
2. Oversees the science of all nursing research activities within designated area of responsibility.
3. Designs research/outcome studies to evaluate patient care issues, models of care delivery, products, and/or technology.
4. Collaborates in multidisciplinary research to promote overall excellence in patient care.
5. Contributes to nursing science as a principal investigator of a program of research.
6. Obtains and manages funding to support research initiatives within designated area of responsibility.

Caring Practices

1. Participates in establishing a caring environment for patients, families, and staff.
2. Facilitates development of caring practices by nursing staff through role modeling, teaching, coaching, and/or mentoring.
3. Cares for the caregivers (i.e., helps staff solve problems, conducts debriefing sessions and crisis intervention).

Response to Diversity

1. Role models, teaches, coaches, and/or mentors acceptance of and responsiveness to unique care needs of patients and families.
2. Identifies evolving trends arising from individual differences and initiates an intervention that would accommodate differences.
3. Assists in the design and evaluation of care-delivery models to meet the diverse needs and strengths of patients, families, staff, and system.
4. Assures that all eligible individuals have equal opportunity to participate in clinical research within clinical area.

Advocacy

1. Contributes to staff knowledge of ethical issues common to clinical area and the conduct of clinical research.

2. Contributes to a clinical research environment that promotes ethical decision-making, protection of human rights, and patient advocacy.

3. Facilitates development of nurses' advocacy and moral agency through role modeling, teaching, coaching, and/or mentoring.

Facilitator of Learning

1. Assesses learning needs of staff and provides both formal and informal opportunities to improve staff's research knowledge and evidence-based skills.

2. Collaborates in the development, implementation, and/or evaluation of unit-based and specialty-based competencies.

3. Supports the professional activities of staff and assists them in disseminating their work outside of Children's Hospital.

4. Participates in the academic community (i.e., participating in collegiate programs, precepting students).

5. Advances nursing science through presentations, publications, and involvement in professional organizations.

Collaboration

1. Role models, coaches, teaches, and mentors nursing staff to understand and use clinical research resources and expertise of others.

2. Mentors staff nurses in professional leadership and accountability for evidence-based nursing practice.

3. Maintains collaborative relationships among teams to facilitate intradisciplinary and interdisciplinary practice and research.

4. Leads multidisciplinary teams in developing programs focused on patient care, staff, and/or system issues.

5. Colleague to members of the hospital research community.

Systems Thinking

1. Role models, teaches, coaches, and/or mentors creative problem-solving and utilization of resources among staff.

2. Assumes proactive role in system redesign that supports a safe environment for staff, patients, and families.

3. Anticipates possible consequences of systems change and develops proactive strategies to enhance evaluation.

4. Applies expert knowledge of the system and works with the entire team to optimize patient care delivery and patient safety.

5. Assumes responsibility to build measurement systems to improve patient care.

6. Develops innovative programs to promote evidence-based practice and advance nursing science.

7. Integrates organizational mission, philosophy, and goals in designated program's research agenda and strategic plan.

8. Represents the clinical scholarship agenda of Children's Hospital in multiple venues (area schools and universities, professional organizations).

Using the Synergy Model in a Peer Review Process

Stephanie Packard, RN, ADN

Peer review is the process by which professional nurses evaluate each other's work performance based on established criteria. The process works best in a practice environment that establishes clearly defined standards of practice, provides the necessary education for staff to meet those standards, and holds professional nurses accountable for their individual and collective practice.

Peer review is an annual requirement for every nurse at Children's Hospital Boston (see Box 4.1). The fundamental tenet of peer review is self-evaluation with input from peers. Peer review is a transparent process in which all reviewers are identified. Participants in the peer review process are expected to maintain a safe, confidential, and respectful process that contributes to the professional development of peers and colleagues. The ideal timing for a peer review is before the annual performance evaluation. Feedback is then incorporated and documented as part of the annual evaluation and considered in determining the merit pay raise. Feedback provided to the individual can be an essential tool for a nurse manager, as it provides concrete examples of an employee's performance from year-to-year and over time.

Box 4.1. Peer review policy from Children's Hospital Boston Professional Advancement Committee.
Used with permission.

Purpose

To evaluate nursing practice in relation to professional practice standards and guidelines, relevant statutes, rules and regulations, and the job document. The goal of peer review is to contribute to the professional development of peers and colleagues (ANA Scope and Standards of Practice, 2003b). The nurse owes the same duties to self as to others, including the responsibility to preserve integrity and safety, to maintain competence, and to continue personal growth (American Nurses Association, 2001).

Definitions

Peer Review	Peer review is the process by which professional nurses are evaluated against established standards of practice within their professional setting.
Peer	A peer is a colleague in a setting who is in a position to observe and evaluate a professional nurse's performance.
Peer Review Tool	This is the mechanism used to gather information for writing a peer review. Tools may differ between practice settings and are based on the generic standards in the job document for each defined level of nursing practice.
Job Document/ Performance Appraisal	Written performance criteria/standards describing expectations for each level of practice. **Reviewee** The nurse being reviewed.
Reviewer	A peer participating in the peer review. The reviewer may provide direct or indirect feedback.

Facilitator	The facilitator is a nurse who has demonstrated expertise in peer review and communication skills. The facilitator is responsible for compiling and summarizing feedback for the peer review.
Nurse Coordinator/ Manager/Director/ VP/CNO	This role in peer review provides the climate and supportive elements needed for peer review to succeed.

Critical Elements

- Peer review is an annual requirement for every nurse at Children's Hospital Boston.

- Peer review is completed before the annual evaluation.

- Peer review is incorporated and documented as part of the annual evaluation and considered in determining the merit raise.

- Peer review is facilitated by a nurse who has demonstrated expertise in peer review.

- Peer review is an open process in which all reviewers are identified.

- Participants in peer review adhere to a safe, confidential, respectful process that contributes to the professional development of peers and colleagues.

- The peer review is based on the reviewee's job documents.

Procedure

Resources

- Professional Advancement Committee

- Nursing Administrative Policy

- Personnel Policy and Procedures

Implementation

1. Every nurse is responsible for ensuring that peer review is completed in a timely fashion.

2. Each participant in the peer review process is responsible for the expectations of roles as defined in this policy.

3. Each program is responsible for developing, implementing, and evaluating its peer review process.

Evaluation

Every nurse has a peer review as part of the annual evaluation.

The Professional Advancement Committee will annually evaluate the effectiveness of the peer review process (American Nurses Association, 2003a; American Nurses Association, 2001; Micheli & Modest, 1995).

Model of Care

The professional practice model establishes the framework for the development of practice standards. In addition, the professional practice model serves as the basis of the clinical ladder and the foundation of the professional advancement process. It is essential for staff nurses at all levels of practice to be involved in developing these practice standards and defining the behavioral elements of the clinical ladder. Staff education focuses on embedding the professional practice model into everyday practice. When nurses understand the fundamental concepts of the professional practice model they can use these concepts in everyday practice, for example, when making nurse-patient assignments.

Synergy Model of Care at Children's Hospital Boston

The professional practice model used at Children's Hospital Boston is the AACN Synergy Model for Patient Care™. The Synergy Model describes individual characteristics that each patient and family brings to a health-care situation. Essential nursing competencies are determined by the needs of the patient and family. Eight dimensions of nursing practice span the continuum from competent nurse to expert nurse. These competencies reflect a dynamic integration of knowledge, skills, experience, and attitudes necessary to meet a patient's needs and optimize outcomes. The evolving expertise demonstrated by staff nurses within these dimensions is the foundation of the professional advancement process and the performance for which nurses are held accountable in their annual peer review.

Nursing Responsibilities

Every nurse within the organization is responsible for maintaining the requisite professional practice standards, including adherence to hospital policy and procedures. In addition, each staff nurse is responsible for developing annual goals and evaluating individual progress toward meeting those goals. The principal duties and nursing competencies specified in the nursing job document are assessed annually by individual staff nurses prior to and during their peer review. Annual goals are reassessed throughout the year with a coach/mentor who works closely with the nurse manager to ensure staff goals are measurable and achievable.

Creating a Supportive Environment

For the peer review process to be fair and equitable for all staff, the job document used for the performance evaluation should accurately reflect current nursing practice and levels of performance, and be understood by staff nurses, coaches, and nurse managers.

Job documents are reviewed yearly to keep them current. This is best accomplished through a centralized Professional Advancement Committee that reports directly to the Nursing Leadership Council. Members of the Professional Advancement Committee should include nurses who have intimate knowledge of the performance evaluation process, familiarity with using the job document, and the ability to create a coaching, friendly environment. Providing individual staff nurses with meaningful feedback aimed at improving performance helps to achieve this. Practice settings that foster "real time" feedback to individuals throughout the year are successful in eliminating the fear of negative, meaningless, or unfair peer reviews.

Developing the Process

The Professional Advancement Committee establishes guidelines for how a generic peer review process should be structured, develops ongoing educational strategies to address knowledge deficits, and identifies members of the committee to serve as consultants for programs within the institution.

All practice settings at Children's Hospital Boston are required to establish a yearly evaluation process that requires at minimum:

- All nurses use a peer review process as a component of their annual performance appraisal;
- Each nurse is responsible for identifying professional goals that are measurable and achievable and for developing strategies to meet those goals; and
- The Children's Hospital job document is the basis of the peer review process.

Individualizing the Process

Practice settings can vary greatly within an institution in terms of number of staff, work flow, experience level of nurses, and knowledge regarding the peer review process. Methods for conducting a peer review depend entirely on the practice environment and are, of necessity, subjective. One method of gathering input is to use an evaluation tool or questionnaire that asks questions related to performance expectations. The questionnaire can be completed independently and forwarded to the peer review facilitator. The limitations of this method are that feedback received is only as good as the questionnaire. The most effective method for gathering input for a peer review is when feedback is shared face-to-face. This method gives the individuals collecting feedback the opportunity to clarify ambiguous information and talk with staff during the input collection process. Regardless of the method used to gather and present feedback, peer review is most satisfying and effective for the individual and the staff member when they learn to integrate the constructive feedback presented during their peer review meeting into their daily practice and interactions with colleagues and peers (see Figure 4.1).

In the neonatal intensive care unit at Children's Hospital Boston, all members of the nursing staff are oriented to the peer review process upon completion of orientation. In addition there is an internal Web-based Peer Review Reference Manual for them to use as an ongoing resource when gathering input and preparing for their own review. This manual clearly describes the peer review process and outlines each individual's responsibility.

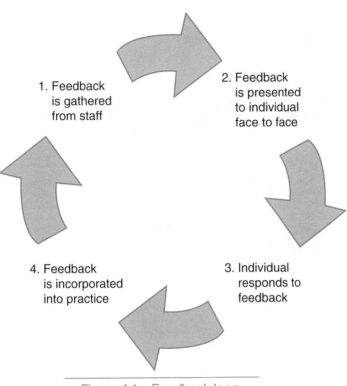

1. Feedback is gathered from staff

2. Feedback is presented to individual face to face

3. Individual responds to feedback

4. Feedback is incorporated into practice

Figure 4.1.   Feedback loop.

NICU Peer Review Process

The NICU Peer Review process consists of the following components (see Figure 4.2):

- Ongoing coaching/mentoring relationship with individual staff
- Document with completed self-evaluation and comments added by the coach/mentor
- Peer review meeting
    - Pre-meeting discussion
    - Meeting
    - Debriefing post meeting
- Meeting with the nurse manager (with final review of the peer review document)
- Document submission to human resources

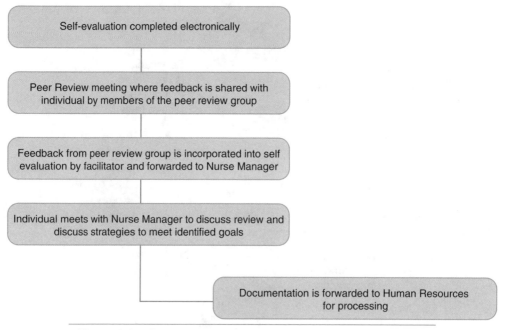

Figure 4.2. Peer review steps, from top to bottom of figure.

Coach, Mentor, Facilitator

Each staff nurse is assigned a coach/mentor through a formal process organized and assessed annually by the nurse manager. Coaches meet periodically with staff, targeting critical times for meetings to assist them with establishing their professional goals, and help them to identify learning needs. The level III coach/mentor also facilitates the staff nurse's annual peer review meeting. While these coaching relationships may vary from individual to individual, based on the needs of each staff nurse, there are several behaviors inherent in the coach/mentor/facilitator relationship.

The level III coach/mentor and facilitator behaviors include:

- Demonstrates expertise and knowledge of peer review process.
- Demonstrates expertise in clear communication.
- Demonstrates expertise in compiling and summarizing feedback.
- Preserves, protects, and enhances the environment that supports caring.
- Creates an environment that fosters mutual respect and professional growth.
- Mentors colleagues in incorporating differences into the provision of care.

- Promotes an environment that recognizes and supports the unique contributions of staff.

- Consistently establishes professional relationships that are characterized by mutual respect.

- Creates and seeks opportunities to coach and mentor and to be taught, coached, and mentored.

In addition, coaches are responsible for completing employee evaluations in a timely manner and forwarding the completed evaluation to the nurse manager for review and edits.

Ideally, each peer review group consists of representatives from all levels of staff—specifically, staff nurse I, II, III. The level III staff nurse also serves as the facilitator of the peer review. The individual being reviewed comes to the meeting with a copy of the completed self-evaluation. Peer reviews are conducted in a respectful, professional manner during work hours. Typically they take about 30-45 minutes and take place about one month before the annual review date. The staff nurse III facilitates the meeting, ensuring that all input is presented in a professional, positive, fair, and understandable manner. Input should be organized and presented using the eight nursing characteristics of the Synergy Model. Before the review meeting, the facilitator meets with the reviewers to strategize on how best to present the input they have gathered. Facilitators should be receptive to the input that has been gathered by the reviewers and not belittle it. The facilitator is responsible for setting the tone of the review. Reviews should be conducted professionally and not casually, like friends chatting. Common themes may be identified from the input that is gathered and presented as strengths and opportunities for growth versus positive and negative.

Peer Review Meeting

The peer review meeting is the forum where all the input gathered is presented to the individual staff member being reviewed. Several times a year the peer review coordinator assigns nursing staff to collect input for a colleague's peer review. The following guidelines are useful for gathering input or providing feedback for a peer review.

Gathering input:

- Interview as many people as possible with varying levels of experience.

- Begin collecting input as soon as you know you are assigned to a review.

- Use the data collection tool (list of eight synergy domains) to help record and organize your input.
- Familiarize yourself with the staff nurse levels of performance (I, II, III).

Providing feedback:

- Feedback should be phrased positively to compliment strengths and identify opportunities for improvement.
- Use the synergy domains of nursing competencies to help stay focused.
- Identify strategies to help the individual accomplish goals.

Employee Self-Evaluation

The individual being reviewed comes to the meeting with the necessary documentation that includes:

- Self-evaluation and yearly summary including accomplishments, contributions, and outcomes that may include, but are not limited to, the following:
    - Meeting attendance record
    - Committee membership summary
    - Participation in projects
    - Promotions
    - Conferences attended
    - Publications
    - Presentations
- A paradigm or exemplar. Staff members who are being reviewed are asked to write an exemplar about an event in the past year that is illustrative of their practice (Benner, 1984).
- Previous year's goals and goals for the upcoming year. Each goal should be measurable and have a strategy for how to achieve it.
- Mandatory requirements may include TB screening, CPR certification, and all requirements that require yearly certification.
- Departmental and unit-based competencies. Includes any department requirement that is renewed and verified annually, such as the use of restraints.

Before the peer review meeting, reviewers gather input and strategize on how best to present what they have collected. The facilitator ensures that the input gathered is presented in a positive, fair, and understandable manner. Basic behavior themes may be identified for the individual from the eight Synergy dimensions. The individual's strengths are identified, and opportunities for growth are discussed. The meeting closes with a presentation of the individual's exemplar. The facilitator then completes the evaluation document by adding a summary of the input from the peer review meeting.

The nurse manager meets with the reviewee soon after the peer review to assess their progress for the year, determine understanding of the input received in the peer review, and identify opportunities for professional growth and development (see Figure 4.3).

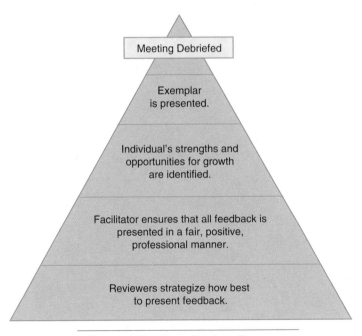

Figure 4.3.   Peer Review Process.

Summary

One of the many reasons peer review is successful in the NICU at Children's Hospital Boston is that expectations are clearly defined and behaviors addressed in real time, not just at the time of the peer review. For peer review to be meaningful and productive for the individual, the philosophy and values inherent in the process must extend to daily nursing practice. Staff nurses are held accountable for their clinical practice; their interactions with patients, families, and staff; and his or her spirit of inquiry on a continuous basis. When honest feedback occurs, individuals are held accountable for their performance. This prevents an individual from hearing feedback in their peer review for the first time. Staff nurses are not only responsible for their own practice; they are responsible for contributing to the success of their nursing colleagues' practice.

The Clinical Nurse Specialist and the Synergy Model

Patricia A. Moloney-Harmon, RN, MS, CCNS, CCRN, FAAN
Kimmith M. Jones, RN, MS, CCNS

The AACN Synergy Model for Patient Care™ has focused mainly on describing the patient-nurse relationship that optimizes outcomes for patients and families; however, it can also be used to elucidate the contemporary practice of the clinical nurse specialist (CNS). Historically, CNS practice has been described as expert clinician, consultant, educator, and researcher. However, these four subroles do not reflect contemporary advanced practice nursing. The role components of today's CNS can be more accurately described by the eight nurse characteristics of the Synergy Model. The CNS has a broad base of knowledge and is required to interact across the organization at all levels. Because of the complex environment in which the CNS practices, three spheres of influence have been articulated that help to explain CNS phenomena of concern (Moloney-Harmon, 1999). The three spheres of CNS influence represent the three consumer groups of patients and families, care providers, and the organization. This broad base allows the CNS to operate on a more global level and influence outcomes on multiple levels.

The History of the CNS

The role of the CNS was developed in the 1960s, although postgraduate education for nurses began in the early 1900s. In the 1970s the American Nurses Association officially accepted the CNS as an expert practitioner and a change agent, requiring a master's degree. The CNS role went through a decline in the 1980s, when many CNS positions were eliminated during the era of hospital restructuring. In that era, there were little data to support the role of nursing, let alone the primarily indirect role of the CNS. In 1995, the National Association of Clinical Nurse Specialists (NACNS) was established with a focus on promoting the CNS (NACNS, 2004; Rouse, in press). The NACNS rearticulated the CNS role as a master's prepared, clinical expert within a specialty area (Zuzelo, 2007). The NACNS also introduced the concept of spheres, which provided a new perspective of CNS practice (NACNS, 1998). This was a move away from the concept of subroles, which were felt to be an inadequate conceptualization of the integrative nature of CNS practice. In addition, the subroles did not acknowledge the effect of CNS practice on outcomes (Fulton, 2003).

Spheres of Influence and the Synergy Model

CNSs intervene and apply influence across three spheres: individual patient/family level, a nurse-nurse level, and a systems level. Each sphere of influence necessitates a characteristic set of competencies to ensure effectiveness. The amount of time a CNS spends functioning in each sphere is determined by the needs of the clinical specialty and the strategic initiatives of the organization in which the CNS works. The patient/family sphere is the foundation for the other two spheres; these spheres are used to advance patient outcomes, quality care, and cost-effectiveness. Within each sphere of influence, the eight nurse characteristics of the Synergy Model represent the advanced level competencies that are necessary for successful CNS practice. Using this model in practice clearly demonstrates the optimal outcomes that result when the advanced level competencies match the characteristics of patients/families, health-care professionals, and the system. The Synergy Model is used by a number of organizations as the basis for the CNS job description because of the link between advanced level competencies and the three spheres as well as its accurate depiction of contemporary practice.

Patient/Family Sphere

The practice base for the CNS is the patient/family sphere. According to the NACNS, outcomes of CNS influence in this domain include: programs of care designed for specific populations; prevention, alleviation, and/or reduction of symptoms, functional problems, or risk behaviors; prevention of real and/or the potential consequences of errors; effective interventions incorporated into practice guidelines; collaboration with team; and the achievement of optimal patient outcomes (NACNS, 2004). Synergy Model competencies within the patient/family sphere of influence that affect patient/family outcomes include:

- Anticipates, synthesizes, interprets, makes decisions, and evaluates responses based on complex, sometimes conflicting sources of data;
- Uses evidence and outcome data to formulate, evaluate, and/or revise policies, procedures, protocols, and standards of care;
- Develops and/or implements a process to ensure that patient/family needs are met with regard to body image, loss, healing, death, and dying/powerlessness; and
- Establishes an environment that promotes ethical decision-making and patient advocacy.

Many studies demonstrate CNS influence in the patient/family sphere. A study conducted by Brooten, Youngblut, Brown, Chin, Finkler, Neff, and Madigan (2001) examined prenatal, maternal, and infant outcomes and cost through 1 year of age using a model of prenatal care for women at high risk to deliver low-birth-weight infants where half the prenatal care was delivered in the home by CNSs. The group cared for in the home had two fetal/infant deaths (control group=9), 11 fewer preterm infants, 77.7% of twin pregnancies carried to term (control group=33.3%), four fewer prenatal hospitalizations, and 18 infant rehospitalizations (control group=24). Prenatal home care provided by CNSs saved 750 total hospital days or about $2,500,000 (Brooten et al.). Deisch, Soukoup, Adams, and Wild (2000) conducted a study examining the use of guided imagery by CNSs in patients who had coronary artery bypass surgery. The study demonstrated that the use of guided imagery reduced pain, fatigue, anxiety, use of opioids, and length of stay and improved patient satisfaction (Deisch et al.). Willoughby and Burroughs (2001) described the foot-care behaviors of diabetic patients who visited a CNS managed foot-care clinic. Their study demonstrated that the clinic patients were more likely to have a foot examination at each visit and to use appropriate foot care practices (Willoughby & Burroughs).

The results of these studies validate the Synergy Model competencies in the patient/family arena. The CNS is demonstrating clinical judgment at an advanced level to ensure positive outcomes for patients and families. Clinical inquiry is made evident by the evaluation of clinical practice and the identification and refinement of innovations for patients and families. The studies show that CNS collaboration with patients and families is essential and that as a facilitator of learning, the CNS contributes to improving patient/family outcomes and quality of care. Caring practices are illuminated as patients experience shorter lengths of stay and fewer complications. Box 5.1 provides an example of the CNS practicing within the patient/family sphere.

Box 5.1. CNS Practice Within the Patient/Family Sphere

LM is an adolescent suffering from complications of end-stage chronic graft versus host disease. She requires continuous renal replacement therapy (CRRT) along with additional interventions, and she is experiencing severe pain. She requests that all life support be removed and that her dog be able to visit her. LM's parents support her but express sadness that she has made this request. The nursing staff wants to meet LM's needs but is uncomfortable with her request to remove life support. They request assistance from the CNS. After speaking to LM and her family, the CNS interprets and communicates the complex patient/family needs to the caregivers. The CNS works with staff, LM, and the family to develop a mutually trusting relationship so that LM can take responsibility for her choices. The CNS helps the staff develop a plan to facilitate the requests so that they are comfortable with the removal of CRRT and the visit of the dog. The dog comes to the unit and spends time with LM; in addition, once CRRT is discontinued, LM's nurses take her to the outside garden. LM dies a few days later and her family states that they feel everything was done to make her death a good one.

The Nurse-Nurse Sphere

A major component of the CNS role is supporting the bedside nurse. The CNS may accomplish this in a variety of ways, including consulting with a nurse at the bedside, teaching a class, or mentoring a nurse through a process. According to the NACNS, the outcomes of the CNS influence in this sphere include the development of knowledge and skills in nursing personnel, along with the provision of state of the art clinical knowledge and skills. In addition, nurses are able to articulate nursing's unique contribution in the care milieu and expected nurse-sensitive outcomes. Nurses resolve patient care issues at the care delivery level, nurses are lifelong learners, and the overall cost of care is decreased through the appropriate use of resources that enhance optimal patient care outcomes (NACNS, 2004). Synergy Model competencies within the nurse-nurse sphere include

- Facilitates development of clinical judgment in health-care team members through role modeling, teaching, coaching, and/or mentoring. Facilitates the development of nurses' caring practices; mentors staff in critiquing literature to determine applicability to practice.
- Cares for the caregivers.

- Contributes to and advances the knowledge base of the health-care community through presentations, publications, and involvement with professional organizations.
- Role models, teaches, coaches, and/or mentors professional leadership and accountability for nursing's role within the health-care system.

Many studies demonstrate the influence of the CNS on nursing and multidisciplinary team practice. Ahrens, Yancey, and Lollef (2003) evaluated the effect of a communication team with a physician and CNS member on length of stay and cost of care for patients at the end of life in an intensive care unit (ICU). The patients who received the communication team intervention had shorter lengths of stay in the ICU and the hospital. In addition, they had lower fixed and variable costs (Ahrens et al.). A pediatric pain management CNS conducted a survey of nurses and was able to identify pain management knowledge deficits, which provided a foundation for education (Manworren, 2000). Dilorio, Price, and Becker (2001) evaluated the first 10 years of a neuroscience nurse internship program developed by CNSs. Results demonstrated satisfaction with both the didactic and clinical content by the internship participants.

CNSs design tools that identify needs or gaps in the knowledge, skills, and competencies of nursing staff to advance the practice of nursing. CNSs are masters at facilitating change. They identify barriers and are able to anticipate consequences of the change that needs to take place. CNSs provide mentorship for the acquisition of new skills and in professional development (NACNS, 2004). CNSs also help staff meet the physical, emotional, and spiritual needs of patients and families and are supported by the CNS in having their own needs met. Through role modeling, teaching, coaching, and mentoring, the CNS ensures the development of all of the Synergy Model competencies in nursing staff. Box 5.2 provides an example of the CNS practicing within the nurse-nurse sphere.

Box 5.2. CNS Practice Within the Nurse-Nurse Sphere

An organization needed to develop an action plan to improve routine pain reassessment throughout the organization. The CNS was asked to spearhead this initiative. The CNS completed a literature search, a survey of other institutions, and an examination of national guidelines to determine best practice. Based on this data, an organization-wide pain strike force was developed with a staff nurse chairperson. The CNS mentored the staff nurse in chairing an organization-wide committee and in communication of the initiative developed by the committee. She also worked with the nurse in data collection and in educating staff. The staff nurse was able to independently assume responsibility for this project within a short time with guidance from the CNS. The nurse received very positive feedback from the large number of people with whom she interacted. The outcome of this program was the successful implementation of a plan to improve the documentation of pain reassessments according to policy in accordance with national standards.

The Systems Sphere

An emerging focus for the CNS is the time spent on system, or organizational, issues. Many organizations use the talents of the CNS to lead organizational change initiatives because of the CNS's mastery of implementing change. For example, the CNS may influence the system through the development of a patient-centered care model for an organization, or the standardization of care for patients within a variety of critical care units. Other examples include the development of an organization-wide approach to decrease or eliminate the number of mislabeled specimens sent to the laboratory, or the development of a clinical pathway for patients with congestive heart failure.

The NACNS has articulated outcomes of CNS influence on this sphere. They include:

- Patient-care processes reflect continuous improvements that benefit the system.
- Change strategies are integrated throughout the system.
- Innovative models of practice are developed, piloted, evaluated, and incorporated across the continuum of care.
- Nursing care and outcomes are articulated at organizational/system decision-making levels.
- Patient-care programs are aligned with the organization's strategic imperatives, mission, vision, philosophy, and values (NACNS, 2004).

As with the other spheres of influence, the Synergy Model describes competencies necessary to achieve the outcomes noted by the NACNS. These competencies include:

- Develop, implement, and evaluate research-based algorithms, decision trees, protocols, and care plans for patients and patient populations.
- Draw on resources including the literature, benchmarking studies, and colleagues to design and evaluate innovations in clinical practice affecting patients/populations and/or systems.
- Contribute to and advance the knowledge base of the health-care community through presentations, publications, and involvement in professional organizations.
- Provide patient/family skills to navigate transitions along the health-care continuum, facilitating safe passage.

Studies that demonstrate the system influence of the CNS exist. Wheeler (2000) conducted a study to determine if patients who received a total knee replacement had better outcomes if a CNS was present on that unit. One hundred sixty-four medical records were included in the study. The researcher found that patients received more nursing care, had shorter length of stays, and had fewer complications on units where a CNS was present (Wheeler).

Alexander, Younger, Cohen, and Crawford (1998) conducted a randomized clinical trial to evaluate a CNS-managed asthma program. Twenty-one patients were enrolled in the study. The researchers found that CNS-managed patients experienced fewer emergency department visits compared to the previous 12-month period before the CNS managed their care.

These studies demonstrate the Synergy Model competencies in the systems arena. Box 5.3 provides an example of the CNS practicing within the system sphere and ultimately the care that is being delivered to patients and families.

Box 5.3. CNS Practice Within the Nurse-System Sphere

An organization decided to forge ahead with a Clinical Decision Support (CDS) initiative. The project consisted of identifying a Clinical Repository, which would be the database for historical and present data related to an individual's care, along with developing the structure of the Clinical Repository, to ensure the system was easy to use and had the necessary information readily accessible to the providers. The CNSs within the organization were involved as consultants in the selection of the Clinical Repository system. Each CNS knew the information within his or her specialty that needed to be available to the providers when the system was accessed. Each CNS participated in a multidisciplinary team to review the repository systems that were being evaluated. At the end of the evaluation, the CNSs submitted their evaluations of the products, which were based on their clinical expertise and the information needs of their areas.

Once the system was selected, a decision was made to proceed with the development and implementation of Computer Provider Order Entry (CPOE). Successful implementation meant that multiple ordersets needed to be developed to reduce the amount of computer entry time for the providers. The CNS group was selected to facilitate the development of the ordersets across a two-hospital health system. The CNS group consisted of seven individuals representing six specialty services: emergency services/ adult critical care, acute care, women's services, children's services, and oncology. The evidence-based ordersets were developed from a system's perspective with involvement from both organizations. Each CNS was responsible for the development of the ordersets within his or her specialty area of practice.

The CNS group began the process by identifying the most common admission diagnoses for their areas of practice. The group consulted with clinical resource management (CRM) to identify these diagnoses. CRM provided the CNS group with a report that listed the most common admission diagnoses by specialty area. The initial orderset list was developed from this report. The CNS group scoured the literature to identify the best practice related to the diagnoses. National guidelines were reviewed and were used in the orderset development along with the most recent research. Current practice within the organization was evaluated to determine if the organization's processes were congruent with the evidence.

Identifying a structural framework for the ordersets was the next step in the process. The framework, which was developed in collaboration with the physician leaders within the organization, identified the essential elements of each orderset. These elements were attending physician, admitting physician, resident, code status, patient care, medications, respiratory therapy, laboratory, diagnostic tests, and consults. Each orderset would identify the most appropriate order within each category.

The CNS drafted all of the ordersets using the framework. A select group of expert physicians were identified and used to review the drafts. Their recommendations were reviewed and incorporated into the ordersets. A broader audience of physicians was used to review the next draft. The ordersets were presented to the Medical Executive Committee (MEC) for final approval once consensus was reached. The ordersets were forwarded to the Information Technology (IT) department once MEC approved the final version. IT was responsible for building the ordersets in the system. The CNS reviewed the work of the IT department to ensure the electronic version of the orderset matched the paper version.

Once the CPOE program was implemented, an orderset review process was developed and put into place. The CNS is the central person to facilitate the development of newly identified ordersets and the revision of existing ordersets. Existing ordersets are reviewed annually.

The orderset development process demonstrates the enormous impact the CNS can have on the system/organization. This process required the CNS to function within the system sphere. The CNS needed to evaluate practice within the organization, determine best practice, and navigate the system to develop ordersets that were comprehensive, multidisciplinary, and promoted the best care for patients and families. A great amount of skill was needed in the area of organizational change and communication to accomplish this monumental task.

Patient Safety

CNSs are uniquely positioned to create a safe environment for patients and families. They are leaders in addressing and resolving safety issues for patients and families. The CNS's goal of ensuring optimal patient outcomes is synonymous with creating an environment of safety (Phillips, 2007). A compelling patient safety issue that has mandated CNS attention is health-care acquired infections, such as central-line infections. This issue has been identified as a major concern across the nation in all patients from neonatal to geriatric (Gerberding, 2002). The Centers for Disease Control and Prevention's (CDC's) National Nosocomial Infections Surveillance (NNIS) system has reported a high number of nosocomial infections from hospitals around the country (CDC, 2003). These infections led to increased hospital costs, morbidity, and mortality (CDC). In 2004, the Joint Commission on Accreditation of Health Care Organizations (JCAHO) added health-care acquired infection to its National Patient Safety Goals (JCAHO, 2004).

A CNS practice group undertook this problem in its institution. The hospital's infection control department reviews all positive blood culture results. The department then examines the patient record to determine if the patient meets the NNIS criteria for central-line-associated bloodstream infections. Data are reported monthly to the ICU multidisciplinary committee and quarterly to the NICU and pediatric multidisciplinary committees. The CNS cochairs these multidisciplinary committees with a physician colleague. Based on the data that were collected and reported, it was determined that an unusually high rate of central-line infections existed in several of the units. Once consensus was reached that a problem existed, the CNSs led an initiative to perform a root-cause analysis. The root-cause analysis identified issues with central-line insertion and maintenance both at the bedside level and the system level. The examination of system and process issues provided an opportunity to identify those factors that increased the possibility of nosocomial infection. By implementing appropriate interventions, the risk of adverse patient outcomes related to nosocomial infection was reduced.

The root-cause analysis began with direct observation through the development and implementation of a central-line audit tool. The audit tool was developed by determining best practice through literature review. The Centers for Disease Control (CDC) Guidelines for the Prevention of Intravascular Catheter-Related Infections, published in the literature, were used to develop the criteria by which to observe practice (CDC, 2002). These guidelines are the benchmark for central-line insertion and maintenance.

Observation of practice revealed that several of the key guideline recommendations were not being performed in all of the units that were identified as having a high infection rate. Breakdowns in the system that contributed to noncompliance with the current procedure were identified. Based on the results of the root-cause analysis, the procedure was revised based on best practice in the literature. This process involved both clinical judgment and inquiry because this was truly a case of developing, implementing, and evaluating research-based recommendations for patients who require central lines. The process also required an appropriate response to diversity on two fronts. Age differences needed to be taken into consideration because the patient populations involved both neonatal and adult. In addition, the key stakeholders were a diverse group, so consensus needed to be obtained with a group that had very different opinions.

The next step was development of a multidisciplinary education plan. The education plan consisted of a brief description of best practice, a review of data from the audit summary, and the procedural changes that were being implemented. Procedural changes included strict sterile technique with line insertion with the use of a full body drape, incorporation of the Biopatch® antimicrobial dressing (Johnson & Johnson), and the use of a more occlusive dressing. In addition, a hand hygiene policy was implemented that prohibited wearing artificial nails, which was strongly supported in reports of best practice in the literature (McNeil, Foster, Hedderwick, & Kauffman, 2001).

Implementation of the education plan occurred over a two-week period. The nursing staff was inserviced during change of shift along with one-on-one education for the few who were unable to attend the formal program. The education of the intensivists occurred during their monthly meeting by the medical director of the unit. Residents were educated on an individual basis by the intensivist overseeing their practice along with the inclusion of the information into their orientation manual.

Experience as CNSs has shown that individualizing the approach based on the audience and involving the key stakeholders in implementation are effective in communicating expectations and changing behavior. After implementation of the education and the revised procedure, the audit was conducted again. The results showed a marked improvement in the identified criteria.

Other system issues were identified. One was that the bedside provider did not have all of the equipment available on the unit to meet the criteria that were being required. Changes in the supply cart needed to occur so that a full body drape was readily available for all central-line insertions. Additional supplies to ensure that dressing changes and administration set changes were done aseptically were made available. It was also stressed with the nursing and physician staff that noncompliance with the stated criteria was not an option for the practitioner placing the central catheter. The medical directors were in full support of the initiative and reinforced the importance of notifying them if physicians did not abide by the new standards.

Subsequent reports from the infection control department demonstrated a dramatic decrease in central line infection rates. Through the vigilance of the CNS practice group, the central-line–associated bloodstream infection rate continues to be on the decline. The organization as a whole has progressed from above the 50th percentile to below the 25th percentile over the past four quarters in the category of nosocomial infection. Reinforcement with the nursing staff and the residents who rotate through the units has been one of the keys to success.

The Synergy Model embraces the concept of providing a safe environment for patients and families. Ensuring patient safety is an essential component of the clinical nurse specialist role. Caring practice is a thread throughout the entire patient safety issue. By ensuring patient safety, safe passage occurs for patients and families.

Summary

This chapter demonstrates how the Synergy Model is used by CNSs to influence care within the three spheres of influence. Numerous examples of how the model is used in practice show convincingly that optimal outcomes will occur when there is a match between higher level competencies and the characteristics of patients/families, health-care providers, and systems. Incorporating the model into contemporary practice inspires CNSs to articulate their unique contribution to the health-care system.

Certification and the Synergy Model

Carol Hartigan, MA, RN

The public is bombarded daily with information regarding various types of regulation. Your local home improvement store promises a certified nursery technician to assist you with all of your gardening needs. Advancement in the field of information technology may be enhanced by obtaining a series of certifications. A row of state licenses is prominently displayed at the neighborhood nail salon. We watch tragic docudramas detailing the negative outcomes of patients who were treated by non-board certified plastic surgeons.

A Harris Interactive Poll conducted by the American Association of Critical-Care Nurses (AACN) in 2002 revealed that public awareness of professional certification is growing. Of 1,039 Americans surveyed, nearly 8 of 10 respondents were aware that nurses could be certified, and 9 of 10 respondents stated that they believed that it is very important for nurses who care for critically ill patients to regularly update their knowledge and skills (AACN, 2003).

Certification? Licensure? What's the Difference?

Although registered nursing licensure has existed in the United States since 1903, nursing specialty certification began in 1945 with the certification of nurse anesthetists and grew significantly in the 1970s as nurses began to specialize in the care of specific patient populations. This care requires specific knowledge, skills, and abilities beyond those obtained in generic educational programs and tested at entry level in the RN licensure examination.

Confusion abounds when discussing regulation, with the terms licensure, certification and credentialing often used interchangeably. *Licensure* is the most restrictive form of regulation, and refers to a mandatory governmental process that grants an individual time-limited permission to use a credential and engage in a specific profession. Licensure most often consists of a combination of a prescribed educational process and an assessment component, and offers title protection for those meeting the criteria.

Professional certification has generally been the term used to refer to a voluntary process in which a nongovernmental agency grants an individual time-limited recognition and permission to use a credential. Certification most often consists of a combination of meeting a set of eligibility criteria that may or may not include an educational component and an assessment component. If the certifying organization has trademarked its credential, it may take legal action against individuals using the credential who have not received it though the certification process.

Credentialing is an umbrella term incorporating the concepts of accreditation, licensure, registration, and professional certification (Durley, 2005). To further add to the confusion, there also exists a hybrid between licensure and certification, sometimes referred to as "statutory certification," a form of title protection or alternative to state licensure, in which a state governmental agency uses a certification examination program developed by a nongovernmental organization as a component in the decision to award a credential in its jurisdiction. This practice came into vogue in the 1970s when a large number of allied health professional organizations began to seek state licensure to qualify for reimbursement for their practitioners in the same way that physicians and nurse practitioners were being reimbursed. Due to this increasing pressure, a moratorium on licensure of additional categories of allied health professionals was declared by the United States' Federal Department of Health, Education, and Welfare—now the U.S. Department of Health and Human Services (Shimberg, 2000). Ultimately, decisions about licensure of health professionals are made on a state-by-state basis, and there are wide variations among jurisdictions regarding which professions require licensure. In many states, for example, occupational therapists may not practice without first passing the certification examination offered by the National

Certification Board for Occupational Therapy, while in other states the examination is voluntary.

As the certification entity of AACN, the AACN Certification Corporation has provided comprehensive credentialing programs for generalists and, more recently, advanced practice nurses caring for acutely and critically ill patients since it was established in 1975. The focus of the AACN Certification Corporation Board of Directors is to protect the public through certification and recertification activities. The corporation certifies registered professional nurses in critical care (CCRN®), progressive care (PCCN®), and clinical nurse specialists in acute/critical care (CCNS®). The corporation will relaunch its acute care nurse practitioner certification program (ACNPC™) in 2007. Subspecialty certification examinations are also available in cardiac medicine and cardiac surgery for currently certified nurses.

AACN Certification Programs— High Stakes Testing?

With the proliferation of allied health professional certification programs in the 1970s, the certification industry grew rapidly during the 1980s. As professional certification examination programs matured and wished to enhance their credibility in the marketplace, as well as to decrease legal liability, they began to adopt nationally accepted best practices for evaluation and testing. These standards include the *Standards for Educational and Psychological Testing* (American Educational Research Association, American Psychological Association & National Council on Measurement in Education [APA], 1985), *The Uniform Guidelines on Employee Selection Procedures* (United States Department of Labor, 1978), *The Code of Fair Testing Practices in Education* (Joint Committee on Testing Practices, 1988), and *The Principles of Fairness: An Examining Guide for Credentialing Boards* (Council on Licensure, Enforcement, and Regulation and the National Organization for Competency Assurance, 1993). Additionally, professional certification organizations began to incorporate psychometric standards into their programs to achieve third-party accreditation by entities such as the National Commission for Certifying Agencies (NCCA) and the American Board of Nursing Specialties (ABNS).

Regulatory examinations that limit an individual's opportunity to practice his or her chosen profession are considered to be "high-stakes" examinations. An example of a high stakes examination is the National Council Licensure Examination for Registered Nurses (NCLEX-RN) exam. It is critically important that high-stakes examinations are legally defensible and psychometrically sound to protect the assets of the licensing or certifying organization from legal challenges by unsuccessful candidates.

Regulatory examinations must:

- Be targeted to entry level practice.
- Measure only job-related knowledge, skills, and abilities.
- Require demonstration of competence at the minimum level necessary for safe and effective practice.
- Be psychometrically sound (Zara, 2000, p. 192).

AACN Certification Corporation's CCNS examination is used as a component in advanced practice licensure or designation decisions by more than 30 state boards of nursing, so it may be considered to be a high-stakes examination in those states where APRN designation is required to practice as a clinical nurse specialist. Although the CCRN and PCCN certification examinations are considered to be voluntary, and thus not as "high stakes" as the APRN exams, the growing prevalence of certification bonuses or differentials and the introduction of policies such as unit-based mandatory certification requirements have made the need to achieve specialty certification increasingly important. Additionally, a number of state boards of nursing have introduced continued competence requirements for relicensure, which include current specialty certification as an option to meet renewal requirements. Unsuccessful certification candidates may be more likely to challenge the content or processes of their examination as the outcome becomes more economically important to them. The AACN Synergy Model of Patient Care™ is a crucial component in ensuring the validity and legal defensibility of each of the AACN Certification Corporation examination programs.

Legally Defensible and Psychometrically Sound

The common catch phrase in the regulatory examination community, "legally defensible and psychometrically sound," generally refers to an examination program that meets best practices in standards and processes. Two key elements in psychometric soundness are examination reliability and validity. Reliability refers to the likelihood that a candidate would receive the same results if they took different but comparable forms of the same certification examination on different days, discounting extraneous factors such as fatigue.

Validity of the examination is related to the ability of the instrument to measure what it is intended to measure—that is, the candidate's job-related knowledge, skills, and abilities. Regulatory examinations are primarily concerned with content validity. Scores on credentialing examinations are considered to be related to the knowledge that underlies the critical skills and abilities necessary to perform effectively in practice. Three assumptions are necessary to document the validity of a credentialing examination:

1. There are certain critical abilities necessary for effective performance, and individuals who lack these abilities will not be able to provide safe and effective care.

2. Individuals scoring low on the examination lack knowledge underlying these critical abilities and will not be able to provide safe and effective care.

3. Examinations can be designed to accurately identify the point at which the knowledge, skills, and abilities demonstrated on the examination are most indicative of the candidate's ability to provide safe and effective care (Fabrey, 1996, p. 16).

The first link in the chain of evidence ensuring the job-relatedness of a regulatory exam is achieved by conducting a job analysis of the role to be licensed or certified. A job analysis may also be known as a role delineation study, role validation, study of practice, or other term. A variety of methods may be used to conduct a job analysis, including focus groups, surveys of incumbents in the role, activity logs, or direct observation. Cost, ease, and access to practitioners may determine the method that is chosen for the research. Regardless of the methodology, the job analysis must determine the critical abilities necessary for safe and effective practice. Accreditation standards require credentialing examination programs to conduct job analyses at least every 5 years to maintain the currency of the examination and to ensure public protection.

At this point in the exam development process, we see some divergence in the focus of the professional association and the certification corporation. The role of the professional association is to advance the profession and to set standards for excellence in clinical practice. The intent of the certification corporation in conducting a job analysis is to document the actual practice of competent practitioners as it currently exists, not to analyze practice as we wish it would be delivered and then to develop an examination based on that ideal scenario.

Role of Experts

To determine the critical abilities necessary for safe and effective practice, an expert panel is convened, composed of geographically and demographically representative participants from a variety of practice settings, including large and small facilities, rural and urban sites, teaching and community hospitals. The panelists must be familiar with the competencies required of the group being analyzed. For example, for the CCRN examination, the group members must understand the knowledge, skills, and abilities required of critical care nurses with 2 years, or 1,750 hours of clinical experience. The panel should include representation from members of the group being considered for certification. The panel members draw on their experience as subject matter experts (SMEs) and may review additional sources of evidence to inform their knowledge of current practice such as textbooks, journal articles, practice protocols, and other contemporary sources. If using the survey method, the expert panel develops a job analysis instrument compiled of a listing of essential tasks, components, or other descriptors of the job being analyzed.

Survey Structure

There is considerable debate in the measurement community as to the best format or structure for the job analysis survey. Should the survey be limited to data collection about specific technical procedures? Knowledge of specific patient problems? Critical thinking abilities such as anticipatory planning? Or specific nurse competencies such as recognizing and tailoring caring practices to the individuality of patient and family?

Because of the complexity of acute/critical care patient needs, the AACN Certification Corporation uses a job analysis survey format that combines data collection regarding patient types, technical procedures and processes, and nurse competencies based on the AACN Synergy Model for Patient Care™. Once a draft survey form has been developed, focus panels refine it. Then, other experts in the field review the form to determine if critical components of the job were overlooked or if any of the questions are unclear or confusing, cover outdated practices, or contain regional biases. Finally, a random sample of incumbents in practice is surveyed.

For Synergy Model nurse competencies, nurses indicate what percentage of their time they spend in each of the competencies. Information is solicited regarding the patient types that they care for on a regular basis. For specific performance-related items, incumbents may be asked to rate the frequency and criticality, or importance, of various tasks on the survey. Nurses indicate how often they performed a given activity in the past week or month, and also rate on a Likert-type scale how important it is to know how to perform the activity correctly. Or, they may be asked how much harm it would cause the patient if the task was omitted. Consider activities such as making a bed—it may be performed with high frequency, but cause little harm if omitted. Defibrillation may be rarely performed, but causes great harm if omitted.

Analysis

After the survey has been completed, the practice analysis task force reviews the responses with the assistance of a psychometric consultant to determine the essential knowledge, skills, and abilities required of the nurse to safely and effectively meet the needs of the patient types. Survey results are reviewed thoroughly for consistency, with careful consideration for institutional or regional differences. Compared to the old days of RN licensure examinations, which took place over a 2-day period, today's nursing licensure and certification computer-based examinations are able to make reliable pass/fail decisions based on as few as 60 to 200 items, depending on the technology and psychometrics. There is no room on the examination for "nice to know" content. Each item on the examination is vital in determining whether or not a practitioner should be designated as certified to provide care for an extremely fragile patient population. This concept becomes particularly significant when developing test plans for APRN examinations. The practice analysis task force prepares a summary of recommended test specifications for the examination. The psychometrician provides recommendations regarding percentages of weight for each component of the examination. The comprehensive test plan includes a description of the individual being certified and the eligibility requirements both for initial certification and recertification. The AACN Certification board of directors approves the final plan.

The Synergy Model and Certification

The Synergy Model was first introduced as the framework for the CCRN Test Plan following a 1997 validation study conducted by Professional Examination Services (PES). During this study, three levels of behavioral descriptions were developed for each of the nurse characteristics by the practice analysis task force. Level 1 descriptors were considered to be a "novice" level, level 3 statements were descriptors for the CCRN level, and level 5 were considered to be descriptive of a CCRN with additional years of performance, or an "expert" level. The results of the job analysis supported the applicability of the Synergy Model to nursing practice. In a second study in 1998, designed to augment the test specifications for the neonatal, pediatric, and adult CCRN credentialing programs, CCRNs identified the overall contribution of each of the eight nurse characteristics to optimal outcomes for critically ill patients and their families. Following this study, the content dimensions of the CCRN Test Plan included Synergy Model nurse characteristics, patient care problems, and nursing process categories (Muenzen & Greenberg, 1998).

A content domain is a major category of a test plan or "blueprint." Examples of content domains could include concepts such as nursing diagnoses, patient care problems, Synergy Model nurse characteristics, or the nursing process. As another link in the chain ensuring the job relatedness of the exam, accreditation requirements state that each examination item must be coded to a component of the test plan. Based on the results of the job analysis, each of the content dimensions will have a percentage of weight assigned to it. The examination forms are assembled based on those percentages so that the final exam will represent actual practice as closely as possible. For example, if "patient care problems" is a content dimension, and the job analysis indicated that 28% of the patients that nurses consistently care for have cardiovascular problems, then the final exam form would contain 28% cardiovascular-related items. If another content dimension was Synergy Model nurse characteristics, and on the job analysis nurses indicated that they spent 4% of their time in the facilitation of learning role, one of those cardiovascular items could ultimately be testing "developing a teaching plan for the cardiovascular patient," and be double-coded.

The beauty of the Synergy Model is that it unambiguously defines the minute-by-minute activities of nurses in any setting so that item coding becomes essentially seamless. In 2001, the nursing process content dimension was dropped from the CCRN Test Plan. Not only was it cumbersome to code items in two nursing models, it was difficult to distinguish between items that were testing for assessment abilities and items that were testing for evaluation abilities. Nursing process remains a component of the item writer guidelines, but items are no longer coded for the nursing process content dimension.

The AACN Certification Corporation again contracted with PES in 1998 to conduct a job analysis to guide the development of a clinical nurse specialist (CNS) examination in acute/critical care. That practice analysis task force used the Synergy Model nurse characteristics as the framework in developing the survey, formulating a level 7 to describe behavioral characteristics of the CNS. Again, the research validated the applicability of the Synergy Model to CNS nursing practice. Following this study, the content dimensions of the CCNS Test Plan included Synergy Model nurse characteristics, patient care problems, and the three spheres of influence toward which CNS activities may be directed.

In the fall of 2002, the AACN Certification Corporation board of directors approved a strategy for a comprehensive study of critical care nursing practice from entry level through advanced practice roles. This was a unique project that had not previously been conducted by any specialty organization. A diverse Practice Analysis Task Force was convened to work with expert researchers from PES to develop survey instruments to define practice characteristics of CCRNs, CCNSs, acute care nurse practitioners (ACNPs), and entry-level (less than 1 year of practice) critical care nurses. Later in the process, a group of 1,000 progressive-care nurses were added to the group. Progressive care is the term used to collectively describe areas that are also referred to as intermediate care units, direct observation units, step-down units, telemetry units, or transitional care units, as well as to define a specific level of patient care. AACN recognizes progressive care as part of the continuum of critical care. The goal in adding the progressive care group was to define the characteristics of nurses practicing in progressive care settings, to identify the types of patients cared for in these units, and to delineate the competencies necessary for safe and effective care. Because of the current shortage of critical care beds, patients are often rapidly or abruptly transferred out of critical care to progressive care units, while still requiring a high level of nursing care and vigilance. An important component of this study was to compare the competencies of CCRNs with those of the progressive care nurses. Other goals of the study were to update the CCRN and CCNS examinations.

Again, the Synergy Model served as the framework for this ambitious project. The original nurse characteristics levels 1, 3, 5, and 7 were revised. Level 7 was renamed 7a for CCNS practice, and a level 7b was developed for ACNP practice. These behavioral descriptions were further refined and validated through expert review and focus groups. Other content dimensions assessed in the study included patient care problems and knowledge and skills (procedures and interventions).

Results of the study reflected current practice as predicted by the expert panels and focus groups. The Synergy Model continued to be validated as the underpinning of acute and critical care nursing practice. The revised level 1 through level 7 behavioral descriptions were validated in the study by nurses from entry level through advanced practice roles, including groups that had never been tested or exposed to the model. All advanced practice participants were surveyed using the same instrument, and the results clearly indicated the similarities and overlaps between roles. The progression of practice from novice (level 1) through advanced (level 7) practice roles was validated in 77% of the behavioral statements. The practice analysis task force then forwarded to the nursing community the recommendation of the test service with the new baseline competencies list; the revised behavioral descriptors for performance at levels 1, 3, and 5 of each characteristic; and the expanded list of advanced practice activities for each nurse characteristic for use in the critical care preceptorship process,

The Synergy Model serves the Certification Corporation well in its mission to protect the public by providing examinations that are job related. But in addition to that important function, the model serves another helpful role. The clarity and completeness of the nurse characteristics statements of the leveled Synergy Model provide the item writers and examination development committees with an understanding of the higher cognitive levels that must be tested to determine competency.

Consider a new item writer developing an item on clinical judgment. For an entry-level examination, the writer would be given the following guideline:

The candidate recognizes normal and abnormal assessment findings.

A CCRN item writer who was writing on the same topic would be given this guideline:

> *The candidate collects and interprets complex patient data.*

A CCNS item writer would be given this guideline:

> *The candidate synthesizes and interprets and makes decisions based on complex, sometimes conflicting, sources of data.*

These specific behavioral statements give the item writer clear guidelines as to how specific and complex the question may be and still be fair to the exam candidate.

Since 1997, the Synergy Model has been validated in research as a workable model for acute and critical care by the practicing bedside nurse. It is easily understandable and unambiguous, and supports dissemination of complete information regarding the content of the certification exams as required by fairness standards and accreditation guidelines. The model is intuitive, and the behavioral descriptors are clearly stated. It has demonstrated the ability to adapt to the rapid changes in acute and critical care nursing practice and is applicable to advanced-practice as well as registered-nurse practice.

Implementing the Synergy Model Within a Multihospital System

Chapter 7

Marilyn Cox, MSN, RN, Melanie Cline, MSN, RN, and Kevin Reed, MSN, RN, CNA

Vision and Model for Transformational Change

Implementing the AACN Synergy Model for Patient Care™ has been a truly transformational experience at Clarian Health in Indianapolis, Indiana. Deep transformational change often begins with a catalyst—like a nurse executive who sees the possibilities of the organization in a different way, a more objective way—and with a vision. Dr. Karlene Kerfoot was that catalyst for Clarian nursing. Kotter (1995) has described a vision as something that clarifies the direction in which an organization needs to move. A vision needs to be big enough to encompass the now and the future, and broad enough so that all see themselves as part of that vision. The Clarian nursing vision of "second to none, transforming the lives of our patients and our nurses" provided for us that all encompassing call to action. Our goal was to be a Magnet hospital and a preeminent nursing division that could and would influence nursing practice at a local, regional, and national level.

Not only has this vision deeply changed the level of professional practice, but it has provided incredible growth and excitement for the people working on the project. Implementing the Synergy Model has resulted in our nurses being re-enchanted with nursing. Planning a change of this magnitude is a challenge, and we all felt the importance of what we were trying to accomplish. For guidance, we used Kotter's (1995) framework for leading transformational change. It was from this framework that we found the guidelines that would serve as our road map for using the Synergy Model to transform the care we provided to our patients and re-create an excitement for nursing practice in our organization. There are eight guidelines in this framework: establishing a sense of urgency, forming a powerful guiding coalition, communicating the vision, empowering others to act on the vision, removing barriers, creating short-term wins, consolidating improvements, and institutionalizing new approaches (Kotter). As we take you through our experience, we will refer to these guidelines, as they provided the basis for the strategic and tactical plan for the creation and implementation of the Clarian Nursing Professional Practice Model.

Choosing the Synergy Model

We were in search of a professional practice model that would reshape nursing practice and illuminate all the important contributions of nursing. We were looking for a conceptual framework that would provide a common philosophy for patient care and nurse development in the context of the current challenges in the health-care environment. Guided by the vision of the chief nursing officer, our goal was to establish Clarian as the benchmark for clinical excellence in multihospital systems.

We were compelled by a sense of urgency that was driven by many factors. As a newly merged organization that included three separate hospitals, we needed a unifying vision for shaping our future and ensuring the best possible outcomes for patients and their families, nurses, and the system. The acuity of our patients and the complexity of the work environment demanded a new paradigm that would emphasize patient centrality and create a culture of professional accountability. At the time we began work on the model, our turnover rate was 18%, our vacancy rate was 12%, and we had become dependent on contracted labor to fill core-staffing vacancies. We were spending millions of dollars in contingency staffing resources and special pay programs. We had also just completed a nurse satisfaction survey and the results were sobering, with scores in several areas such as satisfaction with manager/staff relationships, work environment, and ability to practice autonomously, at a 50% satisfaction level. We needed a model that would resonate with nurses and move us to an environment filled with the forces of Magnetism.

Conceptual models are important because they illuminate what is essential or relevant to a discipline (Curley, 2004). While various models have been used to describe professional nursing practice, we chose the Synergy Model, which was originally crafted by a think tank commissioned by the AACN Certification Corporation, the credentialing arm of the American Association of Critical-Care Nurses (AACN), to describe certified nursing practice (AACN Certification Corporation, 1995). The beauty of the Synergy Model lies in its simplicity: It identifies the patient as the central focus, describing the patient's needs and the skills required of the nurse to best meet those needs (Curley, 1998). It provides clear concepts for defining the relationship between nurses and their competencies and the characteristics or needs of patients. Most importantly, it makes sense to nurses because it articulates their unique contribution to patients, each other, and the health-care system.

We began the work of implementing the use of the Synergy Model by focusing on the nurse characteristics. It was our belief that to fully understand and respond to the needs of patients, we first needed to define the competencies nurses required to meet those needs. Coupled with the urgency to respond to our current challenges, we were compelled to raise the bar on professional practice and create an environment that would recognize and reward clinical excellence and leadership contributions. The call for change was clear, and the focus was to be nursing practice. To begin the transformation, it was paramount to focus our efforts entirely on defining what behaviors needed to change and in what way. Our vision of clinical excellence, "second to none," was established, and it guided us as we formed the coalition to propel us forward.

Successful transformations require a powerful coalition that goes beyond the head of an organization. They must include a mass of people, who come together to develop a shared commitment to excellent performance through renewal (Kotter, 1995). For us, building a powerful guiding coalition included identifying key partnerships and assembling a group with enough power to lead the change. We were fortunate to develop a unique partnership with AACN where we became the clinical incubator for the application of the Synergy Model across an entire health system. In addition, consultation with Dr. Martha Curley provided the vital expertise of the model that we needed in the initial phases of development. The structure for leading us into the future included the formation of the Synergy Steering Committee. Members of the committee were recognized leaders in clinical practice, staff development, human resource management, and change agency. Subcommittees with internal experts on all of the nurse characteristics were formed along the way to formulate various components of the model in detail. Through a series of widespread reviews of the work, more than 1,500 professionals from multiple disciplines were included in the coalition. The approach to development of the model became the energy behind widespread communication of the vision driving our work. Everyone involved in the work began to incorporate the vision and strategy into their thinking. Every imaginable vehicle was used to communicate the vision and the strategies for how it would be revealed. Led by the example of the guiding coalition, the transformation had begun.

The Guiding Principles

The primary outcome of our initial work was the development of job documents that recognize, reward, and promote professional nursing practice. The program goals were to articulate professional nursing practice for all Clarian nurses, promote nurse satisfaction, improve recruitment and retention, provide a framework for professional development toward expert clinical practice, and differentiate pay for nursing staff according to the stage of clinical practice and scope of contribution to clinical practice leadership. The articulation of professional nursing practice began with an examination of core beliefs and values about the practice of nursing at Clarian Health. We began with a critical assessment of existing job documents and an analysis of previous clinical ladders that had been used in the institution. We believed we could start from these documents and build a new vision from our current reality.

As a result of this self-examination, we determined the nursing practice at Clarian was not anchored in a nursing theory, model, or framework. Most importantly, the foundation of our practice was not defined by the nurse-patient relationship. As a result of the 1990s re-engineering and work redesign movement, major portions of nursing practice were removed from bedside nursing job documents and the professional nursing practice role at Clarian had begun to unravel.

The previous nursing clinical ladders had failed primarily because they focused on nurse-centric parameters, and nursing could not demonstrate a difference in patient outcomes as a result of the ladder. A culture of "entitlement" had been created in which all nurses believed they deserved to be promoted after 2-3 years of practice. This "entitlement" culture had resulted in an escalation of the cost of nursing without any visible outcomes to patient care or the organization. Given the lack of measurable outcomes, the organization determined there was no return on its investment.

The failure of the clinical ladders had resulted in the development of a single RN job document. The nursing staff felt "victimized" by the loss of the clinical ladder and mourned the loss of recognition experienced with the clinical ladders. We quickly realized that the current reality base was broken beyond repair and could not serve as a jumping-off point. Therefore, the essence of nursing at Clarian Health had to be different from what it had been before. The dialogue that occurred as a result of these deliberations formed the foundation for the rebirth of professional nursing practice based upon a new set of core values and beliefs.

Patient Centrality

This new set of values began with a commitment to anchor nursing practice with the patient at the core and to build practice keeping the patient and nurse relationship as the central focus. The Synergy Model describes the elements necessary to optimize patient care by defining the needs of the patient and matching those needs to the competencies of the nurse (Curley, 1998). The Synergy Model is historically embedded in the practice of nursing as defined by Virginia Henderson (Curley, 2004). Nursing is primarily assisting the individual (sick or well) in the performance of those activities contributing to health or his recovery (or to a peaceful death) that he would perform unaided if he had the necessary strength, will, or knowledge (Henderson, 1960). It is likewise the unique contribution of the nurse to help the individual to be independent of such assistance as soon as possible (Henderson). The Synergy Model was chosen to provide the framework for nursing practice in order to maintain patient centrality as we built the future.

Differentiation

We had experienced the results of having a single job description and learned that nursing practice is not static or fully described by a single role. We believed that nursing practice is differentiated, and in order to recognize the individual contributions of all nurses, the program would reflect this differentiation. The concept of differentiated practice is defined as a philosophy that focuses on the structuring of roles and functions of nurses according to education, experience, and competence (Koerner & Karpiuk, 1994). We embraced the concept of differentiation and chose to create three separate and distinct job descriptions differentiated by stage of practice and scope of responsibility. The description of how nurses advance in their clinical expertise from one level to another is based on Patricia Benner's work *From Novice to Expert* (1984).

Choice

We clearly intended to create personal choices for nurses in selecting their career path, practice level, and level of participation in the leadership of the unit, service, and organization. This core value was an extremely important decision and clearly a departure from our previous culture of "entitlement." Our culture had been one in which nurses felt and behaved as if they were powerless. This sense of powerlessness had to be addressed, and the primary strategy was to build the concept of choice into the core belief system and infrastructure to support this concept in the new model. In the book *Implementing Differentiated Practice*, Koerner and Karpiuk (1994) devote an entire chapter (Chapter 4) to a concept analysis on choice. Through the experience of implementing differentiated practice at Sioux Valley Hospital, the authors had determined choice to be a cornerstone value. When given the chance to participate in making choices, nursing staff members were empowered and proactive (Koerner & Karpiuk). The importance of this concept was significant, as this assumption was built into the job descriptions as a basic assumption that nurses would engage not only in personal choices about career path, but also engage in organizational choice and decision-making to create and sustain a professional practice environment that best supports the care of patients.

Excellence

We were determined to build this new model through a commitment to excellence that would include an evidence-based approach to "raise the bar" and elevate practice to a level never achieved before in our institution (Kerfoot, 2001). We desired a future state in which all practicing nurses would have a multidimensional practice encompassing the eight competencies as defined by the Synergy Model. This commitment to excellence positioned the nursing department for a habitual and perpetual revolution toward excellence and aligned nursing with the vision of Clarian Health to be a preeminent provider of health care.

Sustainability With a Visible Link to Outcomes

As Joyce Clifford, RN, PhD, FAAN, (2004) noted, the challenge for nursing models is to create flexibility in order to respond to the changing context of practice while staying focused on the time-honored essence of practice—the relationship of the nurse with the patient and family. We were fully committed to create a model that would be sustainable over time and that would provide Clarian nursing a strategy for demonstrating the value of nursing's contributions to patient care outcomes and to the organization. This was critical to the long-term viability of the program and would be necessary to demonstrate the value of the program to the organization.

Creation of the Job Documents

The methodology for the creation of the RN job documents required dimension development of each of the eight nursing competencies, the establishment of content validity across all practice areas at Clarian Health, and the development of criterion measures to fully evaluate the behaviors for each of the dimensions.

Dimension Development

Rapid design sessions were planned with the goal of producing a working draft of job behaviors leveled from competent to expert stage, with 4-10 behaviors listed under each stage for each dimension. The size of the team varied depending on the size of the dimension, ranging from 15-25 participants. Each development team included nurses from each of our three hospitals. Representation also included content experts from disciplines outside of the department of nursing. For example, representatives from chaplaincy and social work participated in the development of the caring practice dimension and provided construct validity for the content. All participants were assigned to read articles related to the Synergy Model, Benner's model of novice to expert, and content specific to the area under development.

The one-day rapid design sessions started with an overview of the project, highlights of the Synergy Model, a review of the core values, and the vision for the creation of the job documents. A brainstorming session was held, and all participants suggested ideas for content and behaviors that should be represented in the job document. The ideas were grouped into similar categories, and participants condensed the ideas to those most relevant to the dimension of practice. The work group was divided into three subgroups and assigned a stage of practice: competent, proficient, and expert. Each subgroup was asked to select from the entire list those behaviors that best represented the assigned stage of practice. In addition, they were asked to come to consensus on the work of the other subgroups on the assignment of behaviors per stage of practice. The drafts from the review sessions then underwent an editing process that included review by Melanie Cline and Kevin Reed, cochairs of the job document process, and Martha Curley, AACN consultant. Edited versions were then returned to the design teams for final approval. All eight drafts were developed over a 3-month period.

Content Validation

The edited drafts were posted on each nursing unit for a period of 1 month. Front-line staff were asked:

- Do the behaviors accurately describe the dimension under development?
- Do the behaviors describe the stage of practice?
- Are there missing elements or redundancies?

Participants were also asked to rank the behaviors in order of importance. Participation in the review process was very high, with more than 1,500 respondents.

Criterion Measures

At the completion of this extensive content validation, we began to develop criterion measures for each of the eight nursing dimensions related to each practice setting. The purpose of developing the criterion measures was to give concrete examples of what constitutes meeting a behavior so that performance could be evaluated against the job documents. Criterion measures were developed by staff nurse groups representing inpatient critical care and acute care (pediatric and adult), outpatient, and procedural areas such as radiology and the operating room. This phase of development was completed when consensus was reached on the equivalency of criterion measures across all practice settings.

Development of a Career Advancement Program

The development of job documents that differentiate levels of practice provided the foundation for the development of a career advancement program, which delineates three levels of clinical practice and leadership. We worked closely with the Clarian Human Resources Department and gained acknowledgment that the job documents constituted distinctly separate levels of job performance, and therefore a promotional opportunity. Borrowing from the model of the professional practice of attorneys and physicians, we defined these three levels as associate partner, partner, and senior partner. Our goal was to establish the idea that we were all partners in the work of patient care and that movement along the levels created increasingly more ownership and responsibility for advancing the practice of nursing.

The three stages of practice for our model are competent, proficient, and expert practitioner. Within each of the job documents is a continuum of progressive knowledge and skills that reflect the needs of a particular patient population. This continuum is reflected in each of the levels through the use of defined behaviors designated as primary or secondary. All of the primary behaviors must be demonstrated before application for promotion. The secondary behaviors within each job document provide an ongoing developmental plan for the newly promoted partner and senior partner. They are designed to provide an additional stretch to raise the bar on clinical practice, scope of practice, and leadership competencies. The secondary behaviors must be met within 6 months of promotion.

The *associate partner* is defined as a competent practitioner whose primary focus is on the relationship with the patient. The scope of the associate partner is the work of direct patient care on a designated unit. The associate partner's practice supports the attainment of nurse-sensitive outcomes that result from direct nursing care including rate of adverse events, complication rates, mortality rates, the patient's length of stay, and patient and family satisfaction.

The *partner* has met the expectations of competent practice as outlined in our associate partner job document and has demonstrated significant movement along the continuum of proficient practice. The primary focus for the partner includes both a focus on the relationship with the patient and their nurse colleagues. At this level, the nurse has expanded her or his ability to concentrate on the patient and demonstrates behaviors that optimize outcomes for groups of patients and the practice of other nurses. The partner's scope of practice contributes to advancing the level of practice on a given unit with the special expertise of precepting, mentoring, or taking on specific unit-based responsibilities such as quality or diversity (Cox, 2004). Partners have the ability to influence outcomes at the unit level. Unit outcomes include measures that are specific to the nurse's contribution and may include such items as compliance with evidence-based process measures, improved regulatory compliance, and a reduction of turnover and vacancy rate of nursing staff.

The *senior partner* is capable of advanced practice over a broad continuum. He or she has met the expectations of proficient practice and has begun to practice at the expert level. The senior partner is highly influential at the system level while retaining the focus on the nurse-to-patient, nurse-to-nurse, and nurse-to-unit relationships (Kerfoot & Cox, 2005). Senior-partner expertise is apparent in interactions with individual patients, nurses, and the health-care system. They are capable of leading system-wide change that results in improved outcomes that may include reduction of complications and length of stay of patient populations, improved resource utilization, and an overall reduction of health-care costs.

To fully realize our efforts to advance the professional practice of nurses, we also defined eligibility requirements for promotion between our differentiated levels. Within the model we conceptualized a professional workforce characterized by higher levels of education, specialty certification, and experience. To advance from the associate partner level to the partner level, 3 to 5 years of experience is recommended, certification is required, and a BSN is preferred. To advance to the senior partner level, 5 to 8 years of experience is recommended, and a BSN and continued specialty certification are required. While there is clearly some flexibility in the experience requirements, we wanted to give some guidance to nurses in developing their career path trajectory and realizing their full potential.

In addition to the eligibility requirements, minimal work hour expectations were established to ensure maintenance of clinical expertise and to build in time away from the bedside to maximize contributions. A work commitment of at least 30 hours per week is required for advancement to a partner level and movement to a senior partner level requires a commitment of 36 hours per week. While initially controversial, over time there has been a realization that the work of the partner and senior partner cannot be accomplished without this level of commitment.

The Process for Advancement

Development of the scope of practice and eligibility requirements naturally led to the evolution of a process by which nurses could apply for career advancement. The components of the process were identified and included the nurse's ability to describe an advanced level of practice and provide evidence of contributions in clinical practice and leadership. In accordance with the core value of personal choice, the staff nurse was given responsibility for deciding whether to seek promotion through the program; thus advancement is defined as optional. One of the elements needed to apply for advancement is a discussion with the clinical manager, which triggers a performance review at the current level and prospective review at the level being sought. Once agreement of readiness between the nurse and the manager is determined, the nurse completes an application and develops a professional portfolio. The portfolio includes documented evidence of the scope of practice reflected by professional activities and contributions including committee activities, leadership with various patient care and outcomes initiatives, and process improvement projects. A minimum of two professional exemplars, which describe real nurse/patient relationships and care experiences that the nurse has encountered, provide the basis for evaluating and staging the level of practice as competent, proficient, or expert. Three letters of reference, including one from the unit manager, are also included.

We developed the role of the Synergy coach to help with the development of the portfolio. Each nurse applying for promotion is assigned a coach at the beginning of the application process. Initially, these were individuals involved in the design and implementation of the program who could mentor the nurse through the application process, including the formulation of an exemplar that reflected an advanced level of practice. This model has evolved over time, with partners and senior partners now also mentoring their colleagues in their professional development and the advancement process.

Once completed, the portfolio is submitted to an internal review board for evaluation and decision-making. The review board is made up of professional nurses from all levels in the organization including partners and senior partners. This allows us to incorporate elements of peer review and enriches the professional nature of the advancement process.

Members of the review board have completed extensive training, which enables them to identify aspects of nursing practice and analyze exemplars to determine the predominant stage of practice. The board of review members are also responsible for the validation of the level of time commitment (FTE) and scope of contribution.

Reward and Recognition Through Compensation

We developed a unique compensation program to reward and acknowledge experience, advanced practice, and the contributions nurses make to patients, unit goals, and system outcomes. The goals of the program included the ability to be easily understood, administered, and sustained in financially tough times; to be effective in recruiting and maintaining a competitive base pay; and to provide reward and recognition for individual performance within each job document based on differentiated practice contributions.

Initially this required an extensive review, assessment, and revamping of our entire nursing pay program. One of our goals was to be highly competitive in the local and regional market with base pay rates at the associate partner level. Through this review we found there were large inequities in pay rates according to experience. An additional goal became the correction of these pay inequities that had been created by previous compensation practices and clinical ladder-type programs. As a result, pay adjustments were made to smooth inequities with current staff and a compensation grid was developed to ensure that entry-level rates would be effective in recruitment of new nurses, and that staff would feel valued for their years of experience. This was an early short-term win. When finalized, the grid included steps that moved base pay rates progressively along a continuum rapidly enough to promote retention, while generating satisfaction with nurses with all levels of experience.

The newly engineered salary grid formed the foundation for the development of a compensation model to support the career advancement program. At the partner and senior partner levels, we worked to develop a model that was competitive at the regional and national market with systems having similar models of differentiated practice. Paid in the form of a percentage increase to base pay, our promotional increases include an 8% adjustment to move from associate partner to partner and an additional 12% increase to move from partner to senior partner. Along with the newly designed salary grid, these increases to base pay allow for the integration of both experience and advancement into the overall compensation package. Other pay practices such as preceptor bonuses and charge nurse hourly pay were dropped once a nurse was promoted to the partner or senior partner level as the expectation for performance of these duties was embedded in the job documents. These changes helped in funding for the new compensation program.

To gain approval and consensus around the compensation design concepts, we developed a return on investment proforma. The projected reductions in turnover and vacancy rates and the elimination of high-cost contracted labor and pay premiums allowed us to calculate and present a proposal that actually demonstrated a cost savings from the implementation of the career advancement program. The greater savings, however, would come from the improved outcomes of patients that could be achieved by a higher level of practice.

Infrastructure to Support the Practice Model

It has been said that to "change everything, focus on one thing" and that to "change one thing requires that you change everything" (Shea, 2001, chapter 2). This was how it was with the implementation of our new practice model. As we completed the job documents, it became clear many things needed to be changed and created to support our goal of a pre-eminent nursing practice model. There were also many obstacles to the implementation of the model. There were systems, structures, programs, and policies that did not fit the new vision and in some instances seriously undermined the vision. Most importantly, cultural and value changes were needed to ensure the model would be embraced and succeed.

Culture Change

The approach to the culture change was fairly bold. We were a pretty typical nursing organization, with traditional management approaches and values. Imagine what happens when the nurse executive starts the communication of the vision with town hall meetings of the staff nurses and not the leadership team. A strategy even more bold was to assign the development of the model below the nurse executive level and with the expectation and emphasis that this was going to be a staff-driven process. Our embedded beliefs were challenged, and a movement from management-centric to staff- and patient-centric was required. It was during this time of destabilization of the "old" culture that rapid movement to the "new" was possible. Those working on the project didn't have to ask for permission to create and innovate. They were empowered to act on the vision and encouraged to take risks, develop nontraditional ideas, and access resources needed to support the project. The values supporting the old culture were challenged as well and had to change. These values were reflected in statements like "a nurse is a nurse is a nurse" or "seniority is the most important determinant for pay." These values and paradigms had to be exposed as antiquated and out of step with the vision.

The Nursing Department

Beyond the culture changes, numerous additional changes within the nursing department were required to support the new model. Our orientation program was not aligned with the new nursing competencies that had been identified. Ours, like those of many other organizations, focused on only a few of the eight dimensions of practice. The orientation content was devoid of any focused exposure to caring practices, response to diversity, or systems thinking. Likewise, we did not have a continuing education program that supported the nurse's advancement in assuming more scope in his or her practice. We identified four areas for curriculum development needed to support the model.

Curriculum on the Synergy Model was designed to establish an understanding and knowledge of the organizing framework based on the Synergy Model. The curriculum for practice established content required by the nursing dimensions of practice for each job document. Work was done on curriculum designed to establish competencies in assessing patient needs according to the eight patient characteristics. The curriculum for leadership focused on skills development in coaching and mentoring; skills in creating, supporting and sustaining a shared leadership environment; and skills in focusing on strengths and talent development versus deficit management. For the staff, there needed to be curriculum on how to advance, which included education on the policies and procedures for advancement, evaluating one's own practice, and how to write exemplars. For the designated board of review members, extensive curriculum on the use of hermeneutic phenomenology to interpret exemplars and stage practice was developed based on the work and expert consultation of Dr. Patricia Hooper Kyriakidis.

With the value change to "education matters and more is better," we needed to conduct a workforce analysis. The focus of this analysis was to determine the percentage of the staff who were prepared at the associate and baccalaureate degree levels, as well what percent of a full-time equivalent they were employed. This was important because we wanted to be able to determine how many staff would be affected by the eligibility criteria for advancement. Based on the results of the analysis, and keeping with our guiding principle of choice, we developed a generous scholarship program with the help of the Methodist Foundation and the Riley Children's Foundation, coupled with a partnership with the University of Indianapolis. The scholarship offers an on-site RN-to-BSN program for those who choose to go back to school and exercise their choice to advance in the field.

Shared leadership became a basic tenet for how we conducted business within the nursing department. We established an aggressive time line for all care centers within each hospital and all units within care centers to establish their structure. In addition, several cross-campus shared leadership councils were established. These included Clarian Clinical Practice Council, with staff nurse representatives from each of three hospitals, the Clinical Director Cross Campus, and the Clinical Manager Councils. All leadership job documents were revised using the eight dimensions of practice outlined in the Synergy Model. We believed we couldn't have bedside staff in one framework for practice and management staff in another. Management needed to be as connected to the model as the bedside nurse, and management and leadership functions needed to be framed in the context of the model. Included were the job documents for clinical director, clinical manager, clinical nurse specialist, and clinical educator. We formed cross-campus groups of clinical managers, clinical educators, clinical nurse specialists, and clinical directors, and charged them with revising their job documents according to the Synergy Model. This was hard work. The first drafts were merely the old job statements reorganized under the eight dimensions. It took several iterations before we finally got to job content that was truly synergized. As a result, there were several new foci that emerged as leadership competencies. These included creating and sustaining a professional practice environment, coaching staff nurses in career advancement, and establishing venues for multidisciplinary collaboration and system alignment. This accomplished two major goals. The leadership staff learned and become immersed in the model. They also began to think about the model in terms of what this change meant to them personally. Initially many in the leadership ranks felt this was only going to change things for the nurse at the bedside. It was at this point we began to see more risk taking, nontraditional ideas, and activities being used at the unit level to promote the model and drive program revisions and development.

The Organization

We conducted a thorough stakeholder analysis to provide a basis for design, strategy, and tactics to gain broad-based support. Key to this analysis was not only to identify the investments and interests of each group, but to put these in the context of a return on the investment. This document became one of the key documents and touchstones as we planned for communication presentations. It also kept us true to the vision. Change of this magnitude has to be communicated in such a way to be explicit about the obvious, and at times the not-so-obvious "What's in this for me?" Stakeholders identified were patients and families; the Clarian registered nurse; physicians who used our facilities; the Clarian support departments, including finance, ancillary departments, human resources, and compensation; and the Indiana University School of Nursing.

Communication plans were drafted for each of the stakeholder groups. It was vitally important that the news of the new program and potential associated compensation program come directly from nursing to each group, particularly the ancillary services, versus through the grapevine. Many hours were spent going to each specific group with these tailored communications.

The most difficult of the hurdles was the finance department and senior hospital executives. They were skeptical that nursing could deliver on such a plan in the face of the budget overruns we were experiencing due to high levels of contingency staffing. With provisional approval, key metrics to demonstrate progress were agreed upon. One of the most powerful characteristics of the program for finance was the movement away from the old entitlement programs represented by previous clinical ladders and the development of unit-specific business plans for the numbers of partners and senior partners needed. Although the number of positions at each level varied according to clinical program and patient need, our overall percent of projected distribution at each job level was 65% associate partner, 25% partner, and 10% senior partner. These business plans were submitted as part of the annual budget development for the organization. In addition to the business plan approach to calculating the overall cost, we were diligent about aligning nursing unit and service patient outcome projects with the Clarian Five Year Strategic Plan, so that a clear articulation of the outputs of the program could be expressed. These included reducing length of stay and complications, and improving patient and family satisfaction.

Outcomes

The implementation of the Synergy Model at Clarian Health was a labor of love and required the proverbial village to build and support. The fruits of this labor are now apparent to us, and the potential for greater outcomes is always on the horizon.

- Clarian Health exceeded the Leapfrog Group quality and safety benchmarks in 25 of 27 categories.
- Patient satisfaction scores are the highest ever recorded.
- Nursing certifications have increased from 5% to 42%.
- The percentage of BSN-prepared nurses working at Clarian Health has increased from 40% to 58%.
- Nursing turnover has decreased from 18% to 8%.
- The vacancy rate has decreased from 17% to 4%.

In addition to these concrete measures, we currently have 200 partners and 15 senior partners actively participating in unit and system decision-making about patient care at a level that is unprecedented. There has been a dramatic increase in the number of nursing staff participating and presenting at national nursing meetings, influencing the practice of nursing at the state, local, and national level. Nurse satisfaction, as measured by the National Database of Nursing Quality Indicators RN survey, has steadily increased in areas such as satisfaction with autonomy and participation in decision-making, opportunity for professional development, RN-to-RN interaction, RN-to-MD interaction, professional status, and satisfaction with job. In the fall of 2004, we achieved Magnet designation through the American Nurses Credentialing Center. To date, we have eliminated $25 million in contingency resources.

Lessons Learned

We have learned many things from our experience with the Synergy Model in creating deep transformational change. The creation of a powerful vision that generates excitement about future possibilities and draws others toward a higher order of things was instrumental in leading us forward. The vision has not only led to a new level of professional practice, it has provided incredible enthusiasm for the work that has been completed and the work yet to be done. Without a powerful vision, one that compels people to move to a preferred future, a change of this magnitude becomes just a group of tasks that result in a feeling of drudgery.

At Clarian Health Partners, we started our work with the nurse side of the Synergy Model. This was based on a sense of urgency to build a professional environment that would enable excellence in patient care and optimal patient outcomes. Organizations that have accomplished this work may choose to start their work with the patient side of the model. While either approach can be successful, the decision should be based on a comprehensive analysis of where the greatest need exists and the ability to build a strong guiding coalition around the work.

The strength of the guiding coalition, including diverse representation throughout the system, enables the ability to generate dialogue to bring clarity to the vision. Repetition and discussion in a variety of forums are needed to expose as many people as possible to the ideas and concepts of the proposed changes. In spite of our efforts, we continue to find pockets of people who have not gotten as much information as others. As difficult as it can be to communicate with nurses in a system that has implemented flexible work patterns, we found this to be a vital step to the success of the project.

We also learned that it is important not to underestimate obstacles along the way. Setbacks will occur and should be planned for to avoid regression that becomes counterproductive to moving forward. Remaining flexible and open to the views and opinions of

The Synergy Model in an Ambulatory Practice Setting

Carolyn Hayes, PhD, RN, CNAA

As a relatively new nurse in Chicago, Illinois, I remember a physician intern once wrote an order in a patient record stating "nursing per routine." I remember being amused by the order. Classes, and even whole courses, in graduate nursing programs are dedicated to answering the question "What is nursing?" What exactly did this intern mean? Of course, any nurse would know he was referring to tasks such as vital signs and assistance with activities of daily living. The order was meant to convey that medical judgment determined this patient needed no more or less observation than stated in the unit-based standards developed with an "average" level of assessed need for the patient population routinely admitted to that patient care area.

What the intern did not understand is that nursing is not definable by the tasks he was seeking for his patient, but rather is relational at its core, and impossible to define by tasks. How could he understand that nursing care is planned and implemented considering, but not solely based on, the patient's disease or treatment plan? It is practiced based on individualized patient-specific phenomenon. Therefore, nursing is ontologically impossible to describe as "routine." Nursing exists only when there is a patient with specific needs and a nurse in relationship with him or her. Ideally it exemplifies the premise for the AACN Synergy Model for Patient Care™, when "patients' characteristics drive nurses' competencies" and patients' outcomes are optimized because "patients' characteristics and nurses' competencies match and synergize" (Curley, 1998, p. 64).

I recalled this incident more than 20 years later while serving as part of a small task force charged at Dana-Farber Cancer Institute (DFCI) to decide on a theory or conceptual model to describe nursing practice in an ambulatory clinical setting. The charge was part of our quest for the subsequently attained Magnet™ status designation (American Nurses Credentialing Center, 2003). Already familiar with the Synergy Model, I accepted this conceptual model as a valid mechanism to determine individualized patient care and to describe the clinical, caring, and moral import of nursing practice in the acute care setting from which it was first conceived (Curley, 1998). The question the task force members wanted answered was: Could a conceptualization of practice originated by critical-care nurses adequately portray diverse ambulatory nursing roles? Should this even be considered?

The conceptual model captured the uniqueness of patients, allowing for eight patient characteristics inclusive of physiological, psychosocial, and spiritual characteristics. However, was the environment in this case different enough from the source environment, critical care, to limit application in an ambulatory setting? Smith (2006) praised the inclusiveness and strength of the model by stating, "Each patient is more than the pressing physiological needs that caused hospitalization for the critical illness" (p. 42). But what about patients not in need of hospitalization? Was Curley (1998) right when she stated, "Although the Synergy Model will be used as a blueprint for the certification of acute and critical care nurses, it is conceptually relevant to the entire profession" (p. 64)? Could this model adequately represent our ambulatory practice?

Background

DFCI is a Magnet hospital with patients who span the continuums of ages and stages of treatment. DFCI's Web site states: "The mission of Dana-Farber Cancer Institute is to provide expert, compassionate care to children and adults with cancer while advancing the understanding, diagnosis, treatment, cure, and prevention of cancer and related diseases. As an affiliate of Harvard Medical School and a Comprehensive Cancer Center designated by the National Cancer Institute, the Institute also provides training for new generations of physicians and scientists, designs programs that promote public health particularly among high-risk and underserved populations, and disseminates innovative patient therapies and scientific discoveries to our target community across the United States and throughout the world" (Dana-Farber Cancer Institute, n.d., para. 1). Adult patients at DFCI are treated in 12 specialized care centers, each devoted to a different type of cancer. DFCI also offers comprehensive family-centered services for children with a suspected or diagnosed cancer or who are at high risk for cancer, as well as care for cancer survivors.

Along with the clinics mentioned, DFCI is a hospital accountable for 27 acute care beds under its license. DFCI patients requiring hospitalization are admitted to either Children's Hospital Boston (CHB), pediatrics, or Brigham and Women's Hospital (BWH), adults. The 27 acute-care beds licensed to DFCI are geographically located at BWH. Nursing practice is multiinstitutional. However, the task force charge to find a conceptual model or theory to describe nursing practice at DFCI was directed to focus exclusively on the ambulatory practice environment.

In ambulatory practice, patient relationships develop during intermittent contacts over long periods of time, which is different from patient relationships experienced by nurses who practice exclusively in acute-care settings. It could be argued that this practice is the other anchor point on a continuum from the originators—critical care nurses—of the Synergy Model. To fulfill our mission, nurses at DFCI practice in a variety of roles. Those roles include RNs practicing as nurse practitioners, research nurses, nurse scientists, infusion nurses, nurse educators, nurse managers, nurse executives, and other nursing roles necessary to create and maintain clinical and research infrastructures.

In 2004, the senior vice president for patient care services and chief nursing officer charged the nursing council to select a nursing theory or conceptual model that would describe nursing practice at DFCI. The use of a conceptual model or theory is considered important to facilitate describing, developing, discovering, and evaluating nursing practice. The nursing council consists of nurses from all roles and is directed to provide a working forum for nursing leadership, educators, and staff within the DFCI/CHB, DFCI/BWH cancer programs to 1) identify priorities and develop recommendations for practice and operational policy changes within nursing, 2) integrate the work of all nursing committees, 3) monitor ongoing projects, and 4) communicate activities to front-line staff. This specific charge to the council was to select a theory/conceptual model that described DFCI nursing practice, would facilitate the work of the council, and would communicate the selection and rationale to their colleagues.

The first step in the selection of a theory or conceptual model was to query council members as to how they would describe DFCI nursing practice. This brainstorming session was facilitated by one of the council members, a nurse manager. In the resulting list of descriptors, the values of our discipline and department were evident. The descriptors were clear that nursing practice at DFCI centered on our patients and their unique journeys. Council members described nursing practice at DFCI in relationship terms, not diagnoses or role-specific terms. In fact, what would become evident later was that DFCI nurses provide "safe passage" for their patients based on the unique needs of each patient.

In addition to the descriptors, the previously stated departmental values were reinforced as essential to our practice in our brainstorming session. Those values are that 1) we create an environment of care that is patient-centered and compassionate, inspiring and motivating; 2) we deliver expert clinical care through evidence-based practice partnerships with patients, families, and colleagues; 3) we exhibit our professional commitment through individual integrity, honesty, reflection, and accountability to self and others; 4) we engage in collaborative decision-making, utilizing available data expertise and wisdom of the collective; 5) we are committed to continuous learning and improvement through high spirit of inquiry, innovation and risk taking, mentoring; 6) we demonstrate respect for patients, families, and colleagues through cultural sensitivity, active listening and response, ethical conduct. For me, as someone reasonably familiar with the Synergy Model, the eight nurse characteristics were visible. For example, "high spirit of inquiry, innovation" was nearly the same language as "clinical inquiry or innovator/evaluator."

The next step for the council was to charge a task force, all members of the larger council, to take the descriptors and the already articulated departmental values to examine for a potential fit with existing nursing theories and conceptual models. The task force reviewed a list of nurse theories and how they define nurse, person, environment, and health and the core concepts of one conceptual model, the Synergy Model. Task force members were charged with doing a more thorough analysis of each theory/model and making a recommendation to the task force regarding how that theory/model fits with the list of descriptors and known department values. In addition, the task force had the benefit of narratives from DFCI nurses describing nurse-patient encounters from actual practice. Each member of the task force could articulate his or her personal practice from the conceptual perspective she was asked to represent, but we could not necessarily articulate DFCI nursing practice overall, based on the descriptors from the council, when challenged to do so. The task force decided to forward two vehicles, Watson's Theory of Transpersonal Caring (2001) and the Synergy Model, as seemingly the best to describe this expert, ambulatory, oncology nursing practice in each of the varied roles we represent.

Narratives as a Means to Decide

Two task force members agreed to present the theory and the conceptual model to the council in depth. The presenters had formal academic and/or research experience, as well as practice, with their respective theory/model. In addition to a presentation on the basic tenets of each, a narrative from DFCI nursing practice was read to the council, and the presenters then applied their respective theory/model to the narrative (see Box 8.1).

Box 8.1. Narrative Used to Demonstrate Synergy Model

by Karen Schulte, MSN, APRN, BC, OCN

It was the end of August and I had just returned to work after having some time off when I noticed I had a new patient on my schedule. I started to do my usual preparation pattern, which was to check to see if there were any pathology reports, radiology reports, or dictated notes. In my process, I discovered that she was a brand new patient to the Dana-Farber Cancer Institute (DFCI), and she had recurrent breast cancer. It dawned on me I had met her about 2 weeks ago when radiology staff had called to say they had a difficult intravenous stick they were sending to the infusion room. The patient, Christina, had an appointment later that morning with me.

A few hours went by and the LPN I worked with, Beverly, told me she had put Christina in one of the private rooms that was available. I entered the room to introduce myself and immediately thought of my sister. It was not that she physically looked like my sister; she just happened to be the same age. Christina and I were 5 years apart in age, just like my sister and me. I could not help thinking that she looked like a model who had been plucked from an expensive clothing catalog. Christina was petite, no more than a size 6, and she stood about 5 feet tall. She had big green eyes framed by a bobbed haircut that was kept pulled away from her face with a single jeweled barrette. As she and I spoke, she went about setting up the room to her liking. She had a tote bag, lunch from home, a book, and a player for her music. After she set up the room, she sat down on the bed and began to tell me the story of her breast cancer.

Christina and her family had recently moved to Natick from Vermont. Her husband, Walt, had signed a 2-year contract to do international consulting with a prominent bank. Christina was not happy about leaving the close-knit community of friends she had developed there. Her most impressive concern was leaving her oncologist's office where she was first treated 3 years prior with stage one breast cancer. Her recurrent disease came as a complete shock to her and her husband, as she had participated in an aggressive clinical trial inclusive of Adriamycin, Cytoxan, Taxol, and radiation therapy upon original diagnosis. Her recurrent disease was discovered on a repeat mammogram taken before the family moved from Vermont. Christina described how she was first diagnosed shortly after the birth of Deborah, her second child, who was now 3 years old. Her oldest child, Richard, was now 7 years old.

I reviewed Christina's functional health patterns with her as I did her initial new patient assessment. She was in a good state of health and had no other medical concerns, but I could not help thinking that if I were her right now, I would be a crazy woman. She had moved, left her circle of friends, and now had recurrent disease. Her whole world had been shaken like a snow globe with pieces scattered from Massachusetts to Vermont. Who would support her? Her husband was going to be traveling a lot with his position and was in South America today. I kept thinking about how she told me that her son, Richard, was at one neighbor's house and Deborah was at another playmate's house, so she must have told her new neighbors that she was ill. I admired her candor as she talked about being afraid of the new treatment, and I was thinking to myself how brave she was, as well as serene, when telling the whole story. Had I been in her size 5 shoes, I would have been a lunatic by now, I kept thinking.

She received her first dose of weekly Taxotere, as well as pamidronate, which she tolerated without incidence. Her only complaint was feeling lethargic from the intravenous Benadryl. We arranged a time for her next visit the following week, and I went about my day. For some inexplicable reason, I could not get Christina out of my thoughts. I had not connected with a patient like this in a while. I wondered if I had become too removed and this particular patient was put on my path to stimulate some re-engagement to what I believed to be the core of nursing: caring, empathy, and advocacy. We had chatted about how her daughter, Deborah, loved clothes, just like my two stepdaughters, and laughed over the trips to the mall we relayed to each other about shopping escapades.

Her son, Richard, loved Harry Potter, which my nephew also loved, and she was reading one of the Harry Potter novels with Richard each night before bed. It was uncanny that both our husbands worked at the same bank, too. In a matter of a few hours, Christina got under my skin.

The next week she returned and we chuckled over what had happened when she returned home the day of her first treatment. She had picked up Richard, who complained that he felt sick to his stomach after receiving a bump on his head while playing at the neighbor's house. Christina called the pediatrician, who advised her to take Richard to Children's Hospital to rule out a concussion. She of course just wanted to take a nap after all the Benadryl. Christina then spoke of trying to struggle to tell her father-in-law, who was staying at the house to help her while Walt was away on business, what the situation was, but he only spoke and understood his native language, not English. The real tricks for Christina were trying to stay awake herself and awaken Richard every 2 hours, because he did indeed have a concussion. We laughed at great length over her ability to juggle home and her illness as well as her new surroundings with a sense of humor.

Over the ensuing months, Christina's recurrent disease began to respond to her chemotherapy regimen. She and I would chat each week during her treatment sessions. Christina was reconnecting with friends from college who lived in the Boston area and taking in the sights, which we would discuss at a great length, exchanging recommendations for outings. Literature was one of our other weekly topics of conversation. We shared a mutual love of reading. She had joined a book club in her neighborhood, and we would swap books back and forth. During the holiday season, Christina was very excited. She had her family coming into town in addition to friends from Vermont. Her shopping was all in order, and her house was decorated with all the holiday trimmings. It was a day or two after Christmas that she and Walt came together to the clinic. I had met Walt once during one of Christina's treatments but was surprised to see him bringing her to the clinic in a wheelchair that day. Walt told me she had vomited her breakfast, and they both thought it was a case of nerves because she was to be restaged today. She had come to see me for the placement of an intravenous line—no ordinary feat as her veins were just as petite as she was.

Christina struck me as anxious that day. I tried to reassure her that she needed to practice her deep breathing and maybe listen to her music so she could reduce her anxiety. Suddenly she looked me right in the eye and said, "I don't feel right." Right then, she began to have a seizure. My heart sank and my adrenaline surged. The code team responded quickly, and we got her seizure activity under control. Her oncologist spoke with Walt about the need to do an immediate head CAT scan to rule out metastasis to her brain.

I was devastated and began thinking how just the week before, Richard and Deborah had come to the clinic with Christina and Walt. Christina had talked about how grateful she was for how I had explained to the children what Mommy and I did together every week to control her cancer. They had taken a tour of the unit, met the pharmacists who mixed Mommy's chemotherapy, met the staff who checked her in, and laughed at my Blue Man Group chemotherapy outfit. In a matter of seconds, it seemed that everything had changed for Christina and her family.

Accompanied by Walt, I wheeled her on a stretcher to radiology for the CT scan. Once she was inside the radiology suite with the technicians, Walt fell apart. He began sobbing uncontrollably. He began talking about how excited she was, just like a little child, on Christmas Eve with her family and friends around, and now this had happened. I had visions in my head, but they were not sugarplums; they were of a disease careening off the train tracks, taking my patient and her family along.

The new year started with whole brain radiation for Christina. Since the seizure, she was wheelchair bound and required nearly total physical care. Walt took a personal leave from his position at the bank and was providing the care required at home. Now each week, they came together for her therapy, and I began to establish more of a rapport with Walt. Realistically I knew that I needed to make sure he had a plan for Christina's passing and a good circle of support around him and the children. It was difficult to watch my patient who had been a beacon of light become an invalid from her disease. She was a fiercely independent woman who now had to rely on everyone for the smallest task. She tried to continue to find humor in all of it. When her hair began to regrow, she decided to dye it blond and bought a funky pair of cat-shaped leopard eyeglasses to replace her tortoise-shell pair.

In early spring, her disease stopped responding. She and Walt made the decision to stop efforts to find hope and instead chose comfort. By May, Christina was living in a hospice as the level of care exceeded what Walt could manage at home, as well as what they wanted to expose the children to. She passed away in the middle of the month.

I remember going to her memorial service and being struck not only by the volume of people in attendance for having been in the community so short a period of time, but also by the feeling of hope. Walt delivered a beautiful tribute to his wife. He spoke of her vitality and spunk as well as her commitment to friends and family. He painted a cherished picture of a gracious lady that I had the privilege to know during a very intimate time of her much-too-short life. The service closed with everyone singing Christina's favorite song, which she sang to her children nightly.

Twinkle, twinkle little star
How I wonder what you are
Up above the world so high
Like a diamond in the sky
Twinkle, twinkle little star
How I wonder what you are

All patient and family names have been changed.

The narrative detailed a nurse-patient relationship from start to finish—the patient's entry for recurrent breast cancer treatment up to the patient's funeral. Embedded in the narrative were descriptors of assessing the patient's and her family's changing needs. The author of the narrative, the nurse, knew because of her expertise and clinical judgment that the patient's diagnosis implied a certain trajectory and predictability, and her social status described resource availability. The nurse also described unique contributors, for example, a recent relocation and two very young children, which would threaten this particular patient's resiliency. As the narrative unfolds, it becomes clear that the nurse uses different skills at different times. When the patient becomes physiologically unstable, the nurse clearly prioritizes her clinical reasoning and systems thinking skills over the previously dominant caring practices and facilitation of learning. The nurse, demonstrating a facilitation of learning and caring practices, took two little children on a tour through a pharmacy and infusion unit to see how and where Mommy got her medicine. This same nurse physiologically rescued a seizing patient, showing her clinical judgment/reasoning.

The presenter to the council was also able to pull from other collected narratives to illustrate the application of the Synergy Model to our practice. For example, one nurse performed a literature review, to find a solution for one of her patients with mouth sores resistant to usual interventions. This exhibition of clinical inquiry revealed morphine mouthwash to be the best possible solution. However, she also discovered there are barriers to pharmacies making this mouthwash available. So, the nurse telephoned area pharmacies until one capable of making the compound was found. That is a clear example of systems thinking.

Yet another narrative details the response to diversity and systems thinking that is necessary in certain situations. The research nurse had to ensure continuity of care for a non-English-speaking 5-year-old and her family, who had to leave their home to get their daughter on a life-saving protocol. There are many examples of advocacy/moral agency and collaboration in the narratives. Every narrative, the descriptors, and the departmental values are clear on the essential presence of caring practices.

A close review of the narratives collected to date revealed that the Synergy Model's eight patient and eight nurse characteristics were all present and could provide a full description of the practice. The model facilitates describing why one patient does not get the same nursing care as his or her demographic mirror image, that is, of the same gender, race, age, and protocol. The uniqueness of each patient generates customized nursing practice.

The council was faced with three options: select one of two choices presented, ask the task force to present different models if neither was a good fit, or decide that no theory/conceptual model would be of use. A postpresentation dialogue ensued with a near-unanimous vote to adopt the Synergy Model. The council members felt strongly that the conceptual model with the eight patient and eight nurse characteristics represented our ambulatory nursing practice well.

The council members articulated that the model resonated with their own and observed practice. In addition, CHB, where our pediatric population is hospitalized, currently uses the Synergy Model in its department of nursing. Leadership staff is shared between these two institutions. One nurse executive accountable in both institutions is a council member and was present for the dialogue. She was able to articulate the benefits and relative ease of incorporating this model into departmental and practice initiatives. Since the decision, other DFCI nurses have had an opportunity to react to the selection of the model. Overwhelmingly, when the basic components of the model are presented to the nurses, they respond, "That is exactly what we do here."

Conclusion

The senior vice president for patient care services and chief nursing officer introduced the model to the entire nursing staff based on the recommendation from the council. In addition, copies of Curley's 1998 "Patient-Nurse Synergy: Optimizing Patients' Outcomes" article were made available in each patient-care and research practice area. Curley presented the model to the council. Moving forward with the Synergy Model as our guide to nursing practice and research at DFCI has been exciting. We believe it represents the nurse-patient relationship embedded in the unique journeys of our patients and families. It allows each nurse to define person, environment, health, and nursing as necessary for his/her practice/research environment but still provides language to describe the unique encounters we value. The Synergy Model is currently being embedded in the department of nursing job descriptions at DFCI, an ambulatory nursing practice whose environment may be very unlike the model's critical care origins, but whose nursing practice is equally synergistic.

Karen Schulte MSN, APRN, BC, OCN, who wrote the narrative beginning on page 111, is Research Nurse for Adult Clinical Trials with the Dana Farber Cancer Institute in Boston, Massachusetts.

NOTE

The author would like to acknowledge the following individuals for their contributions to this work: Patricia Reid Ponte, DNSc, RN, FAAN, Susan Bauer-Wu, PhD, RN, Patricia Branowicki, MSN, RN, CNAA, Anne Gross, MS, RN, CNAA, Katherine McDonough, RN, MS, Lillian Vitale Pedulla, RN, BSN, MSN, Elizabeth Tracey, RN, PhD, AOCN, CS, Dinah Collins, RN, BSN, OCN, Susanne B. Conley, RN, MSN, CPON, CNAA, Susan DeCristofaro, RN, MS, OCN, Marsha Fonteyn, PhD, RN, Monica Fulton, RN, BSN, MBA, Suzanne Hitchcock-Bryan, RN, MPH, Karen Polinski, RN, BSN, MEd, Kristin Roper, RN, MS, OCN, Robin Sommers, MS, APRN, BC, AOCNP, Lisa Brennan, RN, BSN, Sandra Kelly, MS, APRN-BC.

Implementing a Synergistic Professional Nursing Practice Model

John F. Dixon, MSN, RN, CNA, BC
Dora Bradley, PhD, RN-BC

The Magnet Recognition Award for hospitals has become a hall-mark of nursing practice excellence (American Nurses Credentialing Center, 2003). Even hospitals that may elect not to seek Magnet status view the criteria as the ultimate benchmark for enhancing professional nursing practice and improving quality outcomes. Because Magnet requires evidence of a professional practice model, many nursing service departments are making a conscious effort to create and implement these models in their organizations. However, Arford and Zone-Smith (2005) pointed out that an organization's commitment to a model may be insufficient to ensure professional nursing practice at the unit level. It is therefore critical to create structures and processes that can translate the model from the organization level into the actual context of the nurse.

Introducing a professional nursing practice model requires an integrated and supporting infrastructure. For the model to have life, it must be threaded throughout both clinical practice and operations. The model should be what we reference against and use as our guide for choices and decisions. All this work does not happen overnight, but rather it is a journey of development, integration, and discovery and represents an ongoing dynamic process. This chapter will discuss our institution's journey to create strategies to operationalize a professional practice model reflecting a strong foundation in the AACN Synergy Model for Patient Care™.

Origins of Our Practice Model

At Baylor Health Care System (BHCS), we had the beginnings of our professional nursing practice model with Synergy as a core foundational piece. The model's development quickly accelerated when Synergy was used as the organizing framework for our new professional nursing advancement program (PNAP). The diligent work done on our PNAP helped us to articulate and differentiate the dimensions of nursing practice in terms of competencies, scope, and outcomes. These efforts created greater clarity for our practice model. As the model continued to evolve, we also felt it was important to include the three defining qualities of professional nursing practice—authority, autonomy, and accountability.

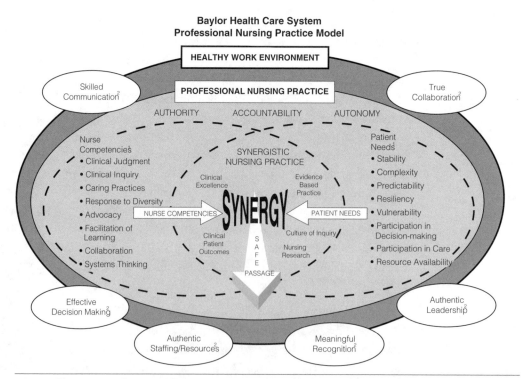

Figure 9.1. © Baylor University Medical Center. Reprinted with permission.

[1]AACN Synergy Model for Patient Care
[2]AACN Standards for Establishing and Sustaining Healthy Work Environments.

Professional practice, however, does not take place in a vacuum. Instead, it occurs within a dynamic organization. The work environment must facilitate and foster professional nursing practice, not create obstacles and barriers. The publication of the *AACN Standards for Establishing and Sustaining Healthy Work Environments* (2005) was a natural fit for the larger context in which our professional practice should occur. By matching patient needs to nurse competencies, we can realize synergistic nursing practice and achieve our outcome goal of safe passage. Building upon Curley's 1998 work, we defined safe passage as "an optimal outcome of nursing. Nurses promote safe passage for their patients by using knowledge of patient needs and the health-care environment to assist them to transition through the health-care encounter without any preventable complications or delay" (Bradley, 2006; see Figure 9.1).

Operationalizing the Model

Leaders must embrace the model and be able to "walk the talk" as a first step. The BHCS professional nursing practice model was adopted by the chief nursing officers across the system. This approval was assisted by the sequencing and timing of having already adopted the PNAP, coupled with the fact that the Joint Commission participated in the national release of the AACN standards for establishing and sustaining healthy work environments, and consultants from Joint Commission Resources, the Joint Commission's education arm, regularly direct clients to the standards. Additionally, the chief nursing officers endorsed a scope of nursing practice that reflected the integration of the new model. Other than the PNAP, which was implemented across most of the health-care system's hospitals, most of the other initial strategies have been implemented first at Baylor University Medical Center, which is a large teaching hospital and the hub of the health-care system. Our efforts focused on creating strategies that would assist in translating the model into the individual nurse's clinical practice.

Initially, the welcome for new hires during general nursing orientation was revamped. Nursing administrators who present this part of the program began to include the model in their presentation with a discussion of its application to professional practice and our definition of safe passage. This introduction allows new hires to hear nursing administration's commitment, "walking the talk," to professional practice and sets the groundwork for continued integration of the practice model that new hires will be experiencing during orientation.

We are continuing to reframe our general nursing orientation so that it solidly centers on nursing practice that promotes safe passage. There are so many things that can be taught or checked off during general nursing orientation, but our goal is to focus our lens on those essential and most vital components that support the nurse in fulfilling our definition of safe passage. Specifically, skills check-offs for equipment, such as infusion pumps, do not just include observation of step-by-step adherence to a procedure, but require the orientee to articulate the rationale for use of safety features in preventing potential adverse events. This concentration will best prepare the nurse to provide interventions and use resources so patients can transition through the health-care encounter without any preventable complications or delay.

Internships have been revised to integrate Synergy Model concepts into their respective curricula. For example, during case studies, questions are posed based on the eight patient needs. For the educators, translating concepts like resiliency or vulnerability into probes was not always easy. As a result, a discussion guide was created (see Figure 9.2). Sample questions were developed for each of the patient needs/characteristics. This resource also has applicability for preceptors who continue on with orientation once the new hire leaves the education department. Nurse managers can select questions from this tool, as well, and use them when rounding on their units to identify key needs of patients.

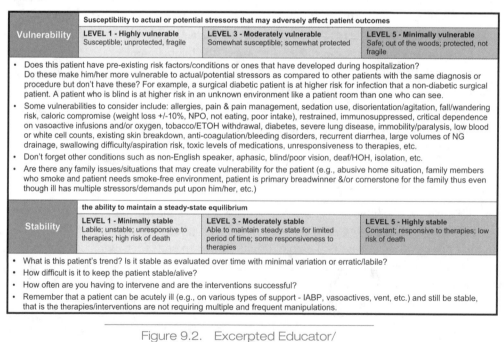

Vulnerability	Susceptibility to actual or potential stressors that may adversely affect patient outcomes		
	LEVEL 1 - Highly vulnerable Susceptible; unprotected, fragile	**LEVEL 3 - Moderately vulnerable** Somewhat susceptible; somewhat protected	**LEVEL 5 - Minimally vulnerable** Safe; out of the woods; protected, not fragile

- Does this patient have pre-existing risk factors/conditions or ones that have developed during hospitalization? Do these make him/her more vulnerable to actual/potential stressors as compared to other patients with the same diagnosis or procedure but don't have these? For example, a surgical diabetic patient is at higher risk for infection that a non-diabetic surgical patient. A patient who is blind is at higher risk in an unknown environment like a patient room than one who can see.
- Some vulnerabilities to consider include: allergies, pain & pain management, sedation use, disorientation/agitation, fall/wandering risk, caloric compromise (weight loss +/-10%, NPO, not eating, poor intake), restrained, immunosuppressed, critical dependence on vasoactive infusions and/or oxygen, tobacco/ETOH withdrawal, diabetes, severe lung disease, immobility/paralysis, low blood or white cell counts, existing skin breakdown, anti-coagulation/bleeding disorders, recurrent diarrhea, large volumes of NG drainage, swallowing difficulty/aspiration risk, toxic levels of medications, unresponsiveness to therapies, etc.
- Don't forget other conditions such as non-English speaker, aphasic, blind/poor vision, deaf/HOH, isolation, etc.
- Are there any family issues/situations that may create vulnerability for the patient (e.g., abusive home situation, family members who smoke and patient needs smoke-free environment, patient is primary breadwinner &/or cornerstone for the family thus even though ill has multiple stressors/demands put upon him/her, etc.)

Stability	the ability to maintain a steady-state equilibrium		
	LEVEL 1 - Minimally stable Labile; unstable; unresponsive to therapies; high risk of death	**LEVEL 3 - Moderately stable** Able to maintain steady state for limited period of time; some responsiveness to therapies	**LEVEL 5 - Highly stable** Constant; responsive to therapies; low risk of death

- What is this patient's trend? Is it stable as evaluated over time with minimal variation or erratic/labile?
- How difficult is it to keep the patient stable/alive?
- How often are you having to intervene and are the interventions successful?
- Remember that a patient can be acutely ill (e.g., on various types of support - IABP, vasoactives, vent, etc.) and still be stable, that is the therapies/interventions are not requiring multiple and frequent manipulations.

Figure 9.2. Excerpted Educator/
Preceptor Guide.
Reprinted with permission from Baylor University Medical Center.

There were varying expectations of the level of performance for new hires when exiting from orientation. Some expect baseline competent performance, while others sometimes expect these new hires to be expert. Our focus has been on "safe and competent," realizing that a person cannot learn every possible detail during orientation. The profile of a safe and competent practitioner is well-defined in the Level 1 definition of the Synergy Model's nurse competencies. Probably what has created some confusion around expectations is not having consistent, well-defined exit goals. The orientee who finishes orientation is a product of the orientation process by both the educator and the preceptor. As such, we should be able to evaluate this "product." The eight nurse competencies at Level 1 have the potential for assisting with this task. We are currently working on an exit-from-orientation evaluation tool. With defined exit goals, the pathway for progression during orientation is much clearer. Plus, the evaluation of this "product," the new hire, may also serve as an evaluation of the quality of the educator and preceptor's work and influence. One of our intensive care units, which is serving as an incubator for best practices, has synergized its specific unit-based orientation processes and materials as a further means to reinforce this approach to practice.

Because Synergy provides an organizing framework for assessing patient needs, it fits well with patient information handoffs. We used Synergy to develop our Professional Exchange Report (PER) guidelines. PER is used for shift change report or when a patient is transferred from one unit to another. Previously, new hires have provided feedback on variability amongst preceptors regarding structure and content of shift reports. While no single process was absolutely wrong, the orientee did not have a clear direction. Orientees did not know whether to create some type of composite, adopt whatever the last preceptor said, or explore and develop their own method through trial and error. This situation pointed out the need for a defined reference or "gold standard." Having such a guideline would help to decrease variability plus provide new hires with a reliable reference tool that guided both structure and content. An introductory script was developed for the patient history, and then the report is based on the eight patient needs. It is not necessary to address every item on the PER guideline, but rather to report only on those items that are applicable to the patient. Three PER guidelines have been created—medical-surgical/telemetry, adult critical care, and neonatal intensive care (see Figure 9.3). Individual feedback from new hires has been positive. They appreciate having a "hard copy" resource that they can reference when they want. Some incumbent staff felt they did not need this guideline, because their perception was that they gave effective reports. However, as managers listened to shift reports by the experienced nurses on their units, they began to realize the structure and content would benefit all nurses' reports.

(Patient Name) _____ **is a** (age) _____ (gender) _____ **in room** (#) _____ **admitted** (#) _____ **days ago on** (date) _____ (*if was via ED note this*) **with** (*chief complaint*) _____. **Attending MD is** (*MD name*) _____.		
Significant/Pertinent/Major medical history includes:	(chronic conditions) (major procedures)	
Since admission, hospital course has included:	(new diagnoses) (major procedures) (complications/problems)	
Patient Needs*	**Content**	**Focus Areas**
Stability	Steady-state equilibrium	• Vital Signs - Patient's Typical Parameters and any deviations • Abnormal Lab/Test/Assessment Results • Meds/Treatments in response to deviations/abnormals
Complexity	Systems Assessment only report findings not within defined limits	• **Neuro** [*altered LOC, disoriented*] • **Cardio/Peripheral Vascular** [*DVT, Pacer, ICD, LVAD, Rhythm, Vasoactive drips*] • **Pulmonary** [*artificial airway, O2 therapy, aspiration potential, swallowing difficulty, chest tube, tobacco usage*] • **Gastrointestinal** [*nausea, tube feedings, ileus, constipated*] • **Genitourinary** [*due to void, dialysis, dysuria*] • **Endocrine** [*diabetic, DFS results*] • **Hemat/Immuno** [*anticoagulated, bleeding disorder, infection, immunocompromised*] • **Integument** [*integrity, incontinent*] • **Musculo-Skeletal** [*immobility, paralysis*]
	[*Selected Key Risks*]	• Vascular Access Devices/IV Therapy/TPN • Incisions/Dressings • Drains/Tubes • Specialty Equipment/Devices • **ISOLATION**
	Psychosocial Needs	• Religious, Spiritual, Cultural Needs
	Pt/Family Dynamics	• Patient/Family Issues
Vulnerability	**ALLERGIES**	• Drug, Food, etc. Allergies
	Pain	• Pain Assessment/Management • PCA/Epidural/PRN Meds • Intrathecal Med – Expiration Time
	Risk Factors (actual or potential stressors)	• Sedation Effects: hypoxia, hypoventilation • Fall/Wandering • Weight Loss +/- 10% • NPO/Not Eating/Poor Intake • Restraints • Immunosuppressed • Others…
	Communication &/or Sensory Limitations	• No English, Aphasic, Blind, Glasses/Contacts, Deaf/HOH, Hearing Aid

Figure 9.3. Excerpted Adult Medical-Surgical/ Telemetry Professional Exchange Report.

Reprinted with permission from Baylor University Medical Center.

Similarly, reports from charge nurse to charge nurse varied across units. A workgroup reviewed this issue and came to consensus on a set of essential content elements. All charge nurses would include these as the core of their report and could add to these based on the unique context of their own unit and patient population. When this consensus list was initially presented in the practice council, the question was raised if these elements could be mapped to Synergy and be consistent with our practice model. Mapping was subsequently done and the charge nurse guideline was synergized. This situation was a good example of staying alert for opportunities to continually introduce and further integrate the professional nursing practice model into operations (see Figure 9.4).

PATIENT NEEDS*	CONTENT AREAS
Stability	Vitals, Labs/Tests ***Codes/RRT Calls**
Complexity	Review of Body Systems Vascular Access Devices/IV Therapy/TPN Incisions/Dressings Drains/Tubes Specialty Equipment/Devices **Isolation** **Medical Alerts**
	Psychosocial Issues
	Patient/Family Issues/Dynamics
Vulnerability	Pain: Assessments, Management, Meds
	Risk & Safety Issues (e.g., Sedation Effects: hypoxia, hypoventilation, Fall/Wandering, Weight Loss +/- 10%, NPO/Not Eating/Poor Intake, Restraints, Immunosuppressed, Aspiration Risk, Paralysis, Errors/Near Misses, Etc.)
	Communication/Sensory (e.g., No English, Aphasic, Blind, Glasses/Contacts, Deaf/HOH/Hearing Aid, etc.)
Participation in Care	Degree of assistance needed
Participation in Decision-Making	Needed Consents/Permits **DNR Status** Advanced Directives/EOL Issues Palliative Care
Resource Availability	Family & other support sources Learning Needed/Ongoing D/C Planning Social Work/Care Coordination
Resiliency	Patient response to illness/coping
Predictability	Course of Illness: **Current Major Nursing Priorities**, Goals of Care yet achieved **Pending** consults, **tests, procedures,** treatments, **surgeries**

Figure 9.4.   Excerpted Charge Nurse Report.
Bolded items are required elements.

One of our programs where Synergy is most widely applied is ASPIRE (Achieving Synergy in Practice through Impact, Relationships, and Evidence), our voluntary PNAP. An advancement program designed to capture and recognize the influence nursing practice has on outcomes is a primary vehicle to translate expectations of the professional practice model. Practice is differentiated into three levels—colleague, mentor, and leader. These levels are differentiated by scope of influence and outcomes of intentional actions at the individual/shift, group/unit, or patient population/system level.

While Synergy elements are woven throughout the program, there are four major categories with distinct mappings to Synergy (see Table 9.1), in addition to the required elements. For each category, the nurse chooses from a number of activities reflecting synergistic practice.

Table 9.1.   **Synergy Correlates.**

Category	Synergy Correlates
Clinical Practice	Clinical Judgment, Caring Practices, Response to Diversity, Advocacy
Leadership	Collaboration, Systems Thinking
Education	Facilitation of Learning
Best Practices	Clinical Inquiry

Reprinted with permission from Baylor University Medical Center.

In addition, the nurse must complete a number of required elements. One of the most exciting of these elements is Linking Nursing Actions to Outcomes for Safe Passage, a clinical narrative. Each nurse, depending on level selected, must describe how their "intentional" nursing actions created safe passage for a patient during an encounter (colleague), a patient across their stay (mentor), or for a population of patients (leader). Through this activity, we have seen nurses move from seeing their actions as "calling the doctor" to applying specific nursing actions to decrease pain for the patient, or extending their assessment to identify how a mother's nutritional status was impacting her breast milk and compromising her infant's life. These examples are truly capturing how a specific nurse's competency when linked to patient needs creates synergy and results in safe passage. Some have said it is the first time that they have taken the time to look at their professional practice and the unique contribution it makes.

Another opportunity presented itself when a system-wide nurse manager survey was being developed. The purpose of this survey was to collect information to accurately describe the current nature, scope, and span of the nurse manager's role. Traditional quantitative measures, such as the size of a unit and number of direct reports, were part of the emerging set of questions. The strict focus on numbers led to a discussion that those measures did not accurately represent the unit. There seemed to be an inherent assumption that the higher the number, the greater the complexity. For example, a unit with 60 beds was more complex than a unit with 30 beds. However, it was noted that if the 30 beds composed a new unit and the 60 beds a well-established unit, it may be that the 30-bed unit has far greater needs and thus may require more nurse manager resources and competencies. So, the focus was directed on how to capture a complete picture. The measures were coupled with the eight characteristics from the Synergy Model, because they can be applied to units and systems. Nurse managers were asked to rate the degree to which their units exhibited the eight characteristics such as stability, complexity, or resiliency. Definitions for each of the characteristics were also included with the survey.

Ongoing work includes inclusion of the practice model's language into such things as policies and procedures. For example, with our Patient Handoff Guidelines policy, the purpose states, "To create safe passage for patients through improved communication effectiveness." As an American Nurses Credentialing Center approved provider of continuing education, we are planning on adopting the Synergy continuing education recognition point (CERP) classification system for all our continuing education programs. By using this classification, staff can determine the nature and scope of their ongoing education choices. We too can evaluate if we are providing diverse offerings, and not just focusing on classic content such as pathophysiology. Hopefully we can revise our job descriptions and performance evaluations to bring them into alignment with Synergy.

What is so nice about Synergy is that most of the differentiating criteria among levels 1, 3, and 5 of performance have already been defined, based on actual studies of practices. Level 1 represents competent practice, level 3 is certified practice, and level 5 is expert practice. These levels would align well with a performance grading system such as good, excellent, and distinguished performer. Probably the most important factor is being continually mindful and aware of opportunities when they present themselves for further integration of the model and the Synergy concepts. We must be careful not to develop tunnel vision and just focus on current projects already underway.

Table 9.2. Synergy CERP.

Category A	Clinical Judgment
	Clinical Inquiry
Category B	Caring Practices
	Response to Diversity
	Advocacy
	Facilitation of Learning
Category C	Collaboration
	Systems Thinking

Some Lessons Learned

We have found that sometimes the word "model" or the picture of the model itself seems to generate in people feelings of discomfort. Such feelings seem similar to ones described by individuals when talking about grand nursing theories from school, as many could not link these directly to practice and thus could not integrate them into their individual practices. A similar phenomenon is observed when the word "research" is used to discuss evidence-based practice. Also, some of the terms in Synergy do not have relevance or personal context for nurses. For example, resiliency may not be something with which nurses can readily identify, so translation is required. Asking questions such as, "How well does your patient rebound from setbacks such as a drop in blood pressure or dizziness when sitting up on the side of the bed?" and, "Does this situation pass quickly or does it require some type of intervention by you to help the patient?" can help staff quickly understand and identify with these situations. This method of exploring practices assists with "backing into" the Synergy Model and helps staff to understand the eight areas of patient need.

When presenting the practice model, a better approach is to start with a discussion about practice. Ask individuals how they approach their practice, how they know what to do, and what organizing framework they use. Sometimes the answer is, "I just take care of my patients," which prompts the question, "How do you go about that?" Such questions typically open the discussion of what nursing practice is, something many have not thought about, given the rapid-fire pace of today's health-care environment. If, as nurses, we cannot clearly articulate our unique contribution to creating safe passage for patients, then how can we expect to be valued? Such discussions often begin with individuals citing various psychomotor tasks, but through continued dialogue the autonomous practice of nursing begins to evolve. From medication administration skills, staff begin to identify nursing interventions, and descriptions of nursing begin to emerge. These descriptions address areas such as assessment, teaching, and evaluation based on unique patient needs. Explorations and discussions such as these help to create linkages to the eight nurse competencies and eight patient needs of the Synergy Model.

As these are adult learners, it is important for staff to understand and see the relevance to their practice. Describing how Synergy evolved from, and is grounded in, studies of actual bedside practice helps fulfill this expectation and assists with clarifying its direct applicability to practice. Additionally, many staff plan on taking CCRN or PCCN certification exams. The exam's blueprint uses Synergy as its framework. Using and applying Synergy as part of practice on a daily basis should better prepare an individual for these certification exams.

Given the predominance of the medical model in health care and an increasing focus on medical practice quality indicators, nurses can unknowingly slip into a biological framework. For example, shift reports may be reduced to a physiologic body systems report. While this information is important, it fails to address the definition of nursing practice: "The protection, promotion, and optimization of health and abilities, prevention of illness and injury, alleviation of suffering through the diagnosis and treatment of human response, and advocacy in the care of individuals, families, communities, and populations" (American Nurses Association, 2004a, p. 7). By using Synergy, the nurse looks at the complete patient and fulfills this accountability.

Enhancing Clinical Reasoning With Undergraduate Students

Chapter 10

Sonya R. Hardin, RN, PhD, CCRN, APRN-BC

The basic goal in nursing education is to facilitate learning through critical thinking skills (Simpson & Courtney, 2002). Teaching or precepting undergraduate nursing students requires the use of effective teaching strategies. Nurses today must possess strong clinical reasoning and clinical inquiry to ensure safe care. Hence, this chapter will describe the use of integrating methods such as the Outcome-Present State-Test (OPT) model, concept mapping, and the AACN Synergy Model for Patient Care™ to enhance clinical reasoning in the care of patients and families. This strategy will be referred to as enhancing clinical reasoning with undergraduate students.

Clinical Reasoning Model

Clinical reasoning is the "reflective, concurrent, creative and critical thinking" used in identifying the best nursing intervention for each given clinical situation (Pesut & Herman, 1998, p. 31). Ultimately, faculty members work with students to help them shift from focusing on tasks to clinical decisions and actions for optimizing patient outcomes.

The Outcome-Present State-Test (OPT) has been described (Pesut & Herman, 1998) and used at the University of North Carolina at Charlotte for teaching clinical reasoning to enhance clinical judgment for more than 5 years. The OPT model uses the facts associated with a clinical case, either designed by an instructor or from the clinical arena, as the context for choosing the nursing action most appropriate for patient goals. Such a model provides faculty and students an alternative to the traditional nursing process of assess, plan, intervene, and evaluate.

Students are taught to identify cues and reflect on the patient's present state as compared to the outcome state through continuous reflective practice (Kuiper & Pesut, 2004). Reflective practice is being in the moment of the learning experience and dancing back and forth between the cues, possible choices, and identifying more data points to consider. Nursing students use subjective and objective cues that present in patient scenarios as present state and to identify outcome states. The facts of a patient case are used to frame the context from which clinical judgments are chosen through reflection and decision-making. Nursing actions are chosen to help patients transition from the present state to the outcome state (See Figure 10.1). Clinical judgment becomes nursing action as choices are made.

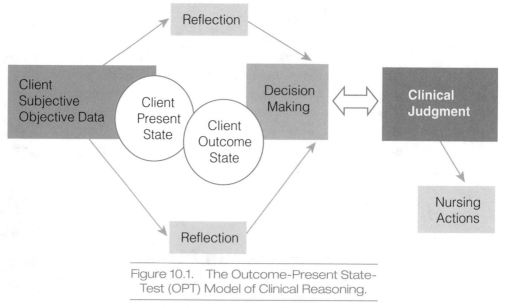

Figure 10.1.   The Outcome-Present State-Test (OPT) Model of Clinical Reasoning.

Based on the work of Pesut & Herman (1998).

While the OPT model provides various thinking strategies such as knowledge work, self talk, schema search, prototype identification, hypothesizing, if-then thinking, comparative analysis, juxtaposing, reflexive comparison, reframing, and metacognitive checks (see

Table 10.1), each student must develop strategies that separate the critical data from the superficial information received during patient assessments, review of the medical record, and review of the most current literature. The student works toward moving the patient toward the outcome state by choosing the best practice. Comparative analysis between the present state and the outcome state is continuously occurring during the time that the nursing student is providing care. These thinking skills are used to develop a graphic depiction, or "concept map," of their thinking and categorization of nursing actions needed in the care of the patient.

Table 10.1. Critical Thinking Strategies Used in the OPT Model.

Knowledge work	Active practice
Self talk	Talking content over in one's mind
Schema search	Using the past to apply to the present
Prototype identification	Use of a model case
Hypothesizing	Identifying possible explanations
If-then thinking	Linking ideas
Comparative analysis	Evaluating competing alternatives
Juxtaposing	Comparing present state to outcome state
Reflexive comparison	Continuously comparing
Reframing	Shifting thinking due to new data
Metacognitive checks	Self-evaluation and self-correction

Adapted from Pesut & Herman, 1998.

Concept Mapping

Concept mapping is "a scheme representing visual knowledge in the form of a hierarchical graphic network composed of nodes and links" (Hsu & Hsieh, 2005, p. 141). Mapping is being integrated into undergraduate curriculums to promote clinical reasoning and evidence-based clinical judgment. This method of analyzing a client situation requires the student to connect the meanings of concepts or nursing actions to capture the entire situation in such a way as to display nursing practice. Information is presented in a logical order and then connected through interconnecting lines to show relationships between concepts and actions. The cognitive processes used in concept mapping are those described in the OPT model. The map can provide a visual picture that shows prior knowledge, experience, and what students are thinking (Hsu, 2004).

Given the complexity of many health-care problems, nursing education must take a new approach to teaching. The use of nursing care plans, while useful at one point in the history of nursing, has become passé. Nursing instruction continues to evolve through the development of different learning strategies. Concept mapping provides the instructor with information to assess student understanding of a clinical case and to clarify students' clinical judgment. The use of clinical reasoning skills, concept mapping, and a theoretical foundation provide a strategy called enhancing clinical reasoning with undergraduate students (ECRUS).

Utilization of Nursing Theory

Nursing theory has been used to shape practice in many nursing schools. Most nursing schools used an eclectic model, while some use grand nursing theories, such as Roy, Roger, Orem, or Neuman. Nursing students need a framework that provides the foundation for structuring and thinking about practice. Proponents of nursing theory believe the best strategy for teaching is through the use of nursing theory. Nursing theory provides the student with focus in the assessment and design of patient-specific interventions.

The theory that can help the student understand the patient and the competencies needed to be a nurse is best found in the Synergy Model. The model is applicable to patients in all settings and at all acuity levels. This model assumes the nurse has the goal of restoring the patient to an optimal level of wellness through the identification of an outcome state. A key focus within the Synergy Model is the integral interconnectedness of the patient and nurse characteristics that, if aligned appropriately, can restore the patient to an optimal level of health (Curley, 1998). The characteristics of the patient and nurse should be considered in the design of patient care. This model is used to enhance clinical reasoning and clinical judgment in a variety of patient settings.

Orientation to the Synergy Model

An overview of the model provides the students with the basic information of the framework and allows the student to ask questions regarding application to practice. The concepts of the model are the eight nurse and eight patient characteristics. These should be fully described so that a clear understanding occurs. When teaching the model, the instructor should describe each characteristic and provide the student with an application in order to facilitate an understanding of the framework for complex patients that are critically ill (Hardin & Kaplow, 2004).

For example, the concept of resiliency is defined as the patient's capacity to return to a restorative level of functioning. Resiliency is accomplished through the use of compensatory mechanisms such as when a patient has low hemoglobin, the heart will beat faster to circulate blood in a manner to deliver an adequate amount of oxygen to the tissue. Resiliency can be demonstrated through case presentations (Kaplow, 2003). Students need to be encouraged to identify the cues that provide data reflecting the patient's level of resiliency. Given the patient's level of resiliency, the student should discuss how each of the eight nursing characteristics must be aligned to support optimal patient outcomes.

Students should be given classroom case examples and then moved to applying the model in the clinical area. Each patient characteristic and nurse characteristic should be analyzed separately, and then in union with each other. Subjective and objective cues should be identified for each characteristic, along with the identification of the level of that specific characteristic for the case. "The level of the characteristic is a useful mechanism in that it allows the student to judge the degree to which the patient is experiencing each characteristic" (Hardin, 2004, p. 3).

A Synergy Model Assessment tool (See Table 10.2) allows students to gather data, organize their thinking, and identify the level at which the patient is presenting each characteristic. This clinical worksheet facilitates critical thinking skills and supports the student in prioritizing the most important cues for each characteristic (Hardin, 2004).

Table 10.2. Synergy Model Assessment Tool for Patient and Nurse Characteristics.

Instructions: Mark an X at the level the client is reflecting each of the characteristics below. Identify supporting data for your assessment.

Patient Characteristic-**Stability**

|———————————————————|
Minimally   Highly

Supporting Data
1.
2.
3.

Patient Characteristic-**Complexity**

|———————————————————|
Highly   Minimally

Supporting Data
1.
2.
3.

Patient Characteristic-**Vulnerability**

|———————————————————|
Minimally   Highly

Supporting Data
1.
2.
3.

Patient Characteristic-**Predictability**

|———————————————————|
Not   Highly

Support Data
1.
2.
3.

continues

Patient Characteristic-**Resiliency**

|————————————————|
Minimally   Highly

Support Data
1.
2.
3.

Patient Characteristic-**Participation in Decision-Making**

|————————————————|
None   Full

Support Data
1.
2.
3.

Patient Characteristic-**Participation in Care**

|————————————————|
None   Full

Support Data
1.
2.
3.

Patient Characteristic-**Resource Availability**

|————————————————|
Few   Many

Support Data
1.
2.
3.

Patient Needs for Each Nurse Characteristic

Instructions: Mark an X at the level of patient need for each of the nurse characteristics.

Nurse Characteristic-**Clinical Judgment**

|————————————————|
Low   High

Support Data
1.
2.
3.

Nurse Characteristic-**Clinical Inquiry**

|————————————————|
Low   High

Support Data
1.
2.
3.

Nurse Characteristic-**Caring Practices**

|————————————————|
Low   High

Support Data
1.
2.
3.

Nurse Characteristic-**Response to Diversity**

|————————————————|
Low   High

Support Data
1.
2.
3.

Nurse Characteristic-**Advocacy**

|————————————————|
Low   High

Support Data
1.
2.
3.

Nurse Characteristic-**Facilitation of Learning**

|————————————————|
Low   High

Support Data
1.
2.
3.

Nurse Characteristic-**Collaboration**   Support Data
                                                1.

|—————————————————————————| 2.
Low   High   3.

Nurse Characteristic-**Systems Thinking**   Support Data
                                                1.

|—————————————————————————| 2.
Low   High   3.

(Hardin, 2004). Reproduced with permission.

Clinical Reasoning

The Synergy Model is essential for facilitating critical thinking skills in baccalaureate education. Patient data can be analyzed through concept mapping or a clinical reasoning web (Pesut & Herman, 1999). In the concept map in Figure 10.2, a student analyzes the patient in relationship to each of the eight patient characteristics surrounding the patient. Within each circle, the student sees a patient characteristic that will need to be completed with subjective and objective cues. A second concept map allows the student to think about the competencies of the nurse in relationship to the patient. The student identifies specific nursing interventions for the patient that are based upon the competencies of the nurse. Data from the patient or case are analyzed and placed in the circle for each characteristic. Then a clinical reasoning web is developed by drawing lines from each characteristic that impacts another characteristic of the patient or the nurse. The patient and nurse concept maps are completed by each student and presented in small discussion groups. Small groups reflect on each characteristic and the cues gathered from the case or the patient (see sample concept maps designed for patient and nursing clinical reasoning webs in figures 10.2 and 10.3).

Faculty should provide the student with a web-analysis rubric to guide the grading of the mapping. Table 10.3 provides a rubric that factors in critical thinking, timeliness, and clarity. Providing a rubric that articulates the scoring for grading a web analysis provides consistency across clinical faculty. Faculty can add more concepts to be measured in the grading of reasoning webs. However, a simplistic design ensures less incongruency between faculty. One point is added when a student provides a reference for an evidence-based article that is relevant to his or her patient and the patient's family. Essentially, a total of 10 points are obtainable with this grid.

Table 10.3. Web Analysis Rubric.

	3	2	1	0
Critical Thinking	Outstanding with superior integration of patient and nurse characteristics, unusual insights, creative and original analysis, reasoning and explanation. The analysis is not just a summary of what was found in the chart, but instead a clear reflection of how the information is interpreted by the student in terms of practice and education is integrated. All material is factually correct, excellent conclusion/integration with sound support. Goes well beyond the minimum required by the assignment.	Good solid analysis that meets minimum required by the assignment. Reasoning and explanations are adequate. The web analysis uses patient data accurately.	Only two of the following are satisfactorily included: 1) use of minimum characteristics, 2) analysis, 3) opinion, and 4) following most of the directions.	A very brief and not necessarily accurate analysis is made or original work is not completed.
Timeliness	The web analysis is completed by the deadline.	The web analysis is turned in one day after the deadline.	The web analysis is 2 days late.	The web analysis is not turned in.
Clarity	The web analysis is clearly written, and contains few grammatical or spelling errors that could undermine clarity.	The web analysis is clearly written.	The web analysis has some clarity flaws but the student's intent is understandable.	Problems with typographical errors, grammatical errors, and so on. These errors interfere with comprehending the intent of the web analysis.
Total Scores				

1 point for an evidence-based article. Maximum number of points obtainable is 10

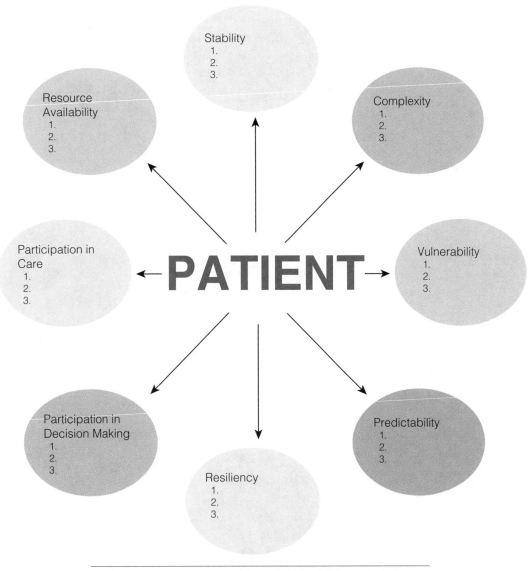

Figure 10.2.   Concept Map of Patient Characteristics.
(Hardin, 2004). Reprinted with permission.

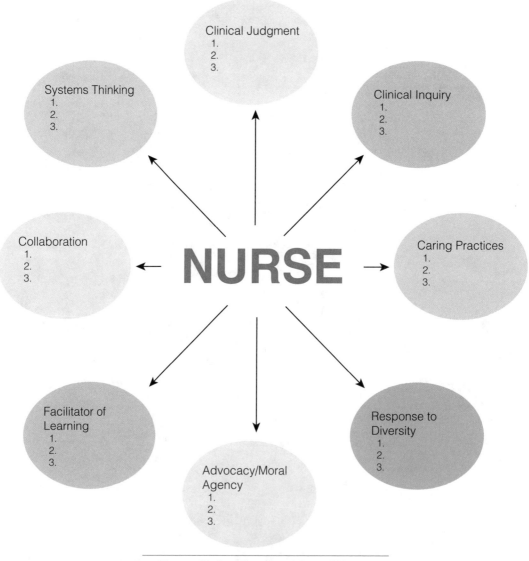

Figure 10.3. Concept Map of Nurse
Characteristics.

(Hardin, 2004). Reprinted with permission.

Student Clinical Assignments

Most undergraduate students spend time in clinical observing, participating in care, and selecting evidence-based interventions through the use of clinical judgment with the oversight of an instructor. The benefit of clinicals is to provide care in a real-life situation. Students are accountable for patient outcomes and responsible for overseeing the care during a typical shift. Before caring for the client, students should have the opportunity to review the medical record and obtain information through a shift report. Students can gain subjective and objective cues from the medical record and through talking with the patient and family. Students begin to interpret data for the Synergy Model from the moment report is given, and continuously throughout the day. The Synergy Assessment tool and clinical concept mapping tools for both the patient and nurse are completed by students and used by instructors to gauge students' knowledge and critical thinking skills. Students draw relational lines between the characteristics and provide a pictorial view of their thinking. The use of different colored pencils facilitates the evaluation of the concept maps by allowing faculty to see how linkages are being conceptualized by students. The Synergy Model clinical concept mapping lays the plan for the nursing interventions to be delivered during the time period that students are overseeing patient care.

The Synergy Model can be used during post-conferences by selecting one characteristic to review in-depth for each patient that the class was assigned. The selection of one characteristic allows students to view the characteristic from multiple patients with a variety of medical diagnoses. Another strategy for applying the model has students present their patient as a case study to the group through describing each patient characteristic along with the subjective and objective cues, the rationale for selection of nursing interventions, and the identified outcome state. Asking other students in the group to provide suggestions can stimulate conversation and further critical thinking. Faculty should ask the student to identify potential complications and describe the cues that would support each potential complication. This level of dialogue can stimulate critical thinking skills. Faculty should also prompt the student to identify previous experiences that helped them to form their clinical decisions. Making linkages with past experiences promotes the use of clinical reasoning. Another strategy to facilitate the understanding of the Synergy Model is to assign students a characteristic to research prior to the next post-conference. Their research should include the latest literature on the concept as it is applicable to a specific medical diagnosis. This information can be shared in a post-conference to help facilitate group learning.

The Synergy Model is useful in guiding students in clinical practice. The model can be combined with clinical reasoning and concept mapping to facilitate clinical judgment. Further development of innovative tools is needed to facilitate learning in the classroom and clinical setting. Undergraduate faculties are challenged to continue the pursuit of creative strategies for teaching and learning to ensure safe practice. Choosing a nursing model such as the Synergy Model can provide guidance to the undergraduate nursing student who has little prior experience with patient care. Historically, most nursing schools have used an eclectic framework, which can be very confusing. The best practice in nursing education is to use a nursing model that can be integrated into classroom and clinical settings to ensure consistency in the delivery of information and reinforcement of content required for knowledge acquisition.

The Synergy Model as a Framework for Nursing Curriculum

Eileen Zungolo, EdD, RN, CNE, FAAN
Maureen Leonardo, MN, RN, CNE, CRNP, BC

The School of Nursing at Duquesne University is using the AACN Synergy Model for Patient Care™ as the framework for the baccalaureate and master's educational programs offered in the school. The purpose of this chapter is to describe the process by which the faculty determined to use this approach, to outline the various internal processes we used, and to summarize how this framework has guided the identification of content and the evaluation of student performance.

The initial interest in the Synergy Model emerged in the fall of 2002, when the faculty of the school began to explore the possibility of developing a critical care focus in the master's degree program. Since the faculty of the school believes that the primary purpose of educational programs is to complement and respond to the needs in the clinical practice arena, we contacted the American Association of Critical-Care Nurses (AACN) to identify experts in both critical care and the educational preparation for that practice. We subsequently invited Ramon Lavandero, director of development and strategic alliances for AACN, and Patricia Moloney-Harmon, author of "The Synergy Model: Contemporary Practice of the Clinical Nurse Specialist," to visit the campus and spend a few days with the faculty as we explored approaches to this new master's emphasis.

The first issue to consider in the planning was to determine the nature of the graduate that we were aiming to produce. There appear to be numerous programs that emphasize the acute care nurse practitioner, while another segment of the nursing education world is committed to the preparation of clinical nurse specialists (CNS) in acute care. We decided to focus on the development of a CNS for a number of reasons, not the least of which is the dearth of leadership in clinical settings and the broad-based concerns expressed by many that the arena of direct patient care is sorely in need of nurses with strong leadership skills.

Once we had decided that the CNS route was our goal, the Synergy Model became increasingly appealing to us as a frame of reference. Our first interest was piqued by the organization of the model, which identifies three spheres of influence: nurse-patient sphere, nurse-nurse sphere, and nurse-system sphere (Moloney-Harmon, 1999). This trilogy of influence spheres appeared to us to ideally reflect the role of the CNS.

In the first instance (nurse-patient), the CNS is an expert in a domain of nursing practice in which the establishment and maintenance of outstanding relationships with patients are vital. In the academic arena at this level, course work focuses on the integration of the skill set required to meet the full range of patient needs as outlined in the model. In the second instance, the focus moves to the nurse-to-nurse sphere. At this level, the central importance is for the CNS to explore ways to maximize the use of nursing personnel and to assist other nurses in developing their competence. The end result of these activities is an enhanced provision of safe care. Within the course work and clinical experiences in the program, emphasis is placed on helping nurses work together in the belief that as nurses grow in their ability to work together, they advance nursing services for acutely ill patients and their families, thereby enhancing patient safety.

Finally, in nurse-system sphere of interaction, a framework for the analysis of the political, economic, and financial realities of the health-care industry is provided in light of the manner in which these impinge on clinical services.

The use of the Synergy Model also enables attention to the competencies of the nurse in practice and how these interact with the spheres of influence. For example, in the first theory-clinical course combination in the master's program, the focus is on enhancing the clinical competence of the nurse in practice with the attention to the nurse-patient sphere.

In the second series of courses, while continuing to foster the nurse competencies in practice, attention is also directed at the development of the collaborative skills of the nurse to enhance the nurse-nurse sphere of influence.

The final course combination in the specialty courses enables the student to develop strategies for working within systems, including skill in financial planning for safe patient care. The student is still working on the advancement of clinical competence. In addition, the student is developing and evaluating research-based decision trees, protocols, and clinical pathways to improve patient outcomes. Considerable effort is directed to fostering new approaches and innovations in health within an interdisciplinary context.

In addition to this course work specific to acute care, the program of study to earn the master of science in nursing includes core work in nursing theory and research, bioethics, and a clinical core (advanced physical assessment, pathophysiology, and pharmacology). The organization and sequential development of these courses is guided by the Synergy Model, as well. Figure 11.1 summarizes the model.

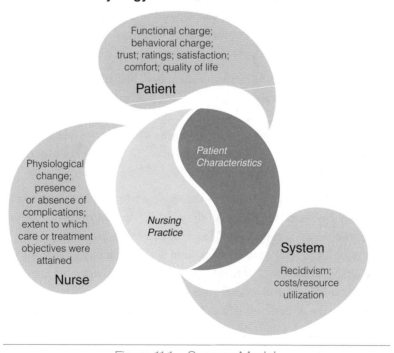

The Synergy Model for Patient Care

Functional charge;
behavioral charge;
trust; ratings; satisfaction;
comfort; quality of life

Patient

Patient Characteristics

Physiological
change;
presence
or absence of
complications;
extent to which
care or treatment
objectives were
attained

Nursing Practice

System

Recidivism;
costs/resource
utilization

Nurse

Figure 11.1.   Synergy Model.
Used with permission. (Curley, 1998).

Baccalaureate Program

Clearly, there is no large leap required to use a model for critical care patients in a specialization program in that clinical domain. However, coincident to the development of the master's program in acute care, the faculty at the school was also reviewing the undergraduate program and exploring various frameworks for utilization with the new curriculum. The faculty began to identify the many aspects of the Synergy Model that were consistent with their values. For example, one element embedded in the Synergy Model that is of critical importance to the faculty is the notion of "safe passage" (Curley, 1998). The responsibility of the nurse to ensure "safe passage" for the patient through all aspects of the health disruption resonated with many beliefs of the faculty. Among the most important to them was the inclusion of end-of-life issues. The faculty at Duquesne University interprets safe passage to mean the provision of support and assistance to the patient and his or her family at all junctures in the illness episode, including through the death process.

Another important dimension of the nurse's competency that was important to the faculty was the characteristic related to moral advocacy. The Synergy Model recognizes and provides for the range of activities and interventions in which a nurse must engage on behalf of the patient and his family, as these relate to representing the interests of the patient. This moral advocacy also assures the patient that his or her values are included in the approaches to care, and that the authenticity of the patient as a unique and valued individual will be respected and supported.

In addition to the above, the faculty of the school had articulated a strong commitment to enhancing the cultural competence of the graduates. Many of the faculty are active members of the Transcultural Nursing Society, and a course in transcultural nursing had long been a staple of the undergraduate and master's programs. Once again there was compatibility between the faculty and the tenets inherent in the Synergy Model in the attention to cultural competence in the nurse characteristic of "response to diversity."

As faculty members began to discuss the approach to patient care inherent in the Synergy Model, they embraced the notion of the need for compatibility between the skills of the nurse and the needs of the patient. However, there was also a commitment among the faculty to develop a program of study consistent with the faculty analysis of the health-care needs of the region; an assessment that led to a need to emphasize the community basis for care and the demands for primary care. Would a framework developed for an acute care setting translate to the other levels of care? How could a practice framework guide curriculum development?

Curriculum Process

We began this curriculum work with a re-evaluation of the philosophy of the faculty about nursing and found that the core competencies of the Synergy Model were consistent with faculty beliefs. As a result, the following statements were introduced to the philosophical statements of the school.

> The faculty believe that there are core competencies that enable a nurse to provide "safe passage" for patients. The core competencies are the basis of the nurse's ability to provide, design, manage, and coordinate caring practices. These core competencies are: clinical judgment, clinical inquiry, caring practices, response to diversity advocacy, facilitation of learning in patients and staff, collaboration, and systems thinking.

The faculty spent a considerable amount of time analyzing the model, specifically assessing the characteristics of the nurse. It was not long before the faculty began to see how these characteristics of the nurse could potentially be used within a curriculum framework as the characteristics of the graduates of the program. We then examined these outcomes and considered how these would be developed over the course of the program of studies. Table 11.1 provides a succinct delineation of the product of that work. Following the table horizontally, the reader can see at each year of the program of study, the level at which the nurse competency is expected to develop. Included at each characteristic are the objectives that provide the learning expectations underpinning the competence. Essentially, this table documents how the competencies of the nurse are developed over the course of the program of study, and clearly demonstrates how these characteristics have been used to guide the progression of content. Essentially the sequential development of these characteristics is leveled across the years of the program and serves as a guide to the delineation of course content. Table 11.2 summarizes the courses at each of these levels, along with broad strokes of the content included. While the progression is succinctly presented, the generation of the table was accomplished over a number of months.

Table 11.1. Development Level and Descriptions of Nurse Competencies

Nurse Competencies	Freshmen	Sophomores	Juniors	Seniors
Clinical Judgment	Introduction to critical thinking/health promotion. Scientific method/logical thinking. Principles of social justice. *Explains the meaning of, and necessity for, using clinical judgment in one's professional role.*	Utilizes the nursing process. Assesses health status. Analyzes critical incidents. *Demonstrates clinical judgment when implementing care for individuals.*	Evaluates one's own clinical decision-making using evidence-based format. Analyzes total plan of patient utilizing CAT. *Analyzes one's clinical judgment when implementing care for individuals, families, and groups.*	Prioritizes nursing interventions for groups of patients. Utilizes principles of delegation and supervision. *Integrates clinical judgment when implementing care for individuals, families, groups, and community.*
Clinical Inquiry	Introduction to evidence-based practice. Introduction to information technologies. *Explains the meaning of clinical inquiry to a profession.*	Examines (EBP) research based knowledge to support nursing interventions in primary care. Utilizes modalities of information technologies in primary care. *Gives examples of research based practice.*	Utilizes (EBP) research based knowledge to support nursing interventions in the acute care setting. Utilizes modalities of information technologies in acute care. *Relates research to clinical practice.*	Evaluates (EBP) research based knowledge to support nursing interventions in acute and long-term care. Utilizes modalities of information technologies in chronic and long-term care. *Engages in the research process to support evidence-based practice.*
Caring Practices	Care of self. Caring processes. *Expresses the importance of caring as related to self and one's profession.*	Initiates caring practices. Incorporates culturally sensitive care. *Initiates caring behaviors.*	Demonstrates caring behaviors to individuals, family, and groups. Assesses one's capacity of caring. *Integrates caring into one's practice.*	Internalizes behaviors of caring practice. Develops an appreciation of diversity of needs for care. *Displays a caring attitude in all aspects of one's practice.*

Nurse Competencies	Freshmen	Sophomores	Juniors	Seniors
Response to Diversity	Introduction to diversity and cultural competence in health-care delivery Assesses self-cultural beliefs. *Describes the meaning of cultural competence.*	Introduction of the impact of racial and ethnic disparities Assesses the role of diversity in health care. *Illustrates examples of culturally competent care.*	Applies concepts of culturally competent care for individuals, family, and groups. *Implements care in a culturally competent manner with all persons.*	Evaluates and develops strategies to promote culturally competent care. *Integrates cultural competence in caring for individuals/families of diverse populations.*
Advocacy/Moral Agency	Introduction to ethics of nursing Introduction to professional nursing Self-advocacy (starts and goes throughout) Self-moral agency (responsibility/accountability) Individual spirituality *Differentiates between the ethical and the legal aspect of one's profession.*	Acts as patient's agent. Differentiates between ethics and law. Develops (introduction to) professional responsibility and accountability and peer accountability. Identifies spirituality in others. *Practices within the ethical and legal framework of one's profession.*	Assesses ethical dimensions of clinical situations and formulates potential interventions. Recognizes an environment that fosters ethical decision making. Recognizes the impact of spirituality on illness. *Engages in ethical decision-making.*	Evaluates ethical and legal dimensions of one's own practice. Evaluates spiritual dimensions of one's own practice. *Justifies one's practice through the implementation of the role of being a moral agent.*
Facilitator of Learning	Describes learning as a factor in health promotion. Examines the teaching/learning process Identifies self-learning styles. Explains the teaching/learning process. *Explores the meaning of patient outcomes and nurse competencies.*	Develops and implements a wellness teaching plan. Implements a teaching plan to promote wellness. *Examines the interrelationship of nurse competencies and patient characteristics to patient outcomes.*	Incorporates teaching as a consistent strategy for acute nursing care. Implements interdisciplinary teaching plans that promote the health of patients, groups, and communities. *Utilizes the unique strengths of the patient characteristics and the nurse competencies to affect patient outcomes.*	Implements a multidimensional educational project. Incorporates the teaching/learning process into all aspects of one's practice. *Evaluates the interrelationship of nurse and the nurse competencies and the patient characteristics to patient outcomes.*

Nurse Competencies	Freshmen	Sophomores	Juniors	Seniors
Collaboration	Group dynamics, principles of cooperation, collaboration and team building *Examines the meaning of collaborative care to one's practice.*	Gathers and shares information with other health-care providers. Cooperates with peers in group endeavors. Identifies roles and functions of other health-care providers. *Describes the meaning of collaboration to health care.*	Identifies strategies for interdisciplinary care and practices. Collaborates with other members of the interdisciplinary team. Cooperates with staff at affiliated clinical agencies. *Engages in collaboration with others in planning and implementing care.*	Evaluates processes of collaboration in the clinical setting. Develops strategies to promote collaboration. Integrates care with other members of interdisciplinary team. *Initiates collaborative efforts for the improvement of care to individuals and for improvement in health-care delivery.*
Systems Thinking	Introduction to health-care systems Introduction to quality management Biological systems Safety systems *Identifies the meaning of a systems thinking approach.*	Assesses the primary health-care access, delivery and finances of the health-care system. Primary care safety Primary care quality *Explains how changes in the system can affect patient outcomes.*	Assesses the acute health-care access, delivery, and finances of the health-care system. Acute care safety Acute care quality *Examines the use of various strategies within the system that can be used to improve patient outcomes.*	Assesses the long-term health-care access, delivery, and finances of the health-care system. Chronic and long-term safety Chronic and long-term quality *Demonstrates the ability to utilize integrated systems analysis for personal and professional navigation of the health-care delivery systems.*

Table 11.2. Curriculum Grid/Program of Studies

Freshmen			Sophomores		
Concepts	**Fall Courses**	**CR**	**Concepts**	**Fall Courses**	**CR**
Self-awareness Personal and professional values (assignments within these first level courses will include community involvement)	**Theology Core**	3	Wellness across the lifespan Wellness across body systems	Human Growth & Development	3
	Life Processes	3		• *Growth & development*	
	Health & Wellness	3		*—Fetal development*	
	• *Definitions of H & W*			*—Reproduction*	
	• *Health Behavior*			*—Death & dying*	
	• *Models of H & W*			*—Developmental*	
	• *Individual & community applications*			*milestones*	
	• *Personal health practices, lifestyle, and behaviors*			• *Cultural variations*	
	• *Health history/personal health appraisal*			• *Role of genetics*	
	• *Cultural rooting*			• *Introduction to family and community assessment*	
	• *Coping strategies*				
	• *Self-esteem*			A & P I	4
	• *Intro to health-care systems as consumers (insurance)*			**Basic Philosophical Question**	3
				Social, Political, Eco Systems	3
	Thinking & Writing Across the Curriculum	3		Principles of Communication	2
	Nutrition for Wellness	3		• *Communications theory*	
				• *Developing therapeutic and culturally competent relations in nursing*	
				• *Conflict and conflict resolution*	
				• *Collaboration concepts*	
				• *Group dynamics*	
				• *Interviewing skills*	
				• *Health history interview*	
				*Synergy in Nursing Practice: Healthy People I	2
				• *Teaching health promotion and wellness, e.g. wellness clinics (prenatal clinics), churches, food banks, senior citizen places, schools, daycare, shelters*	
				• *Evidence-based practice applications*	
		15			**17**

BOLD = University Core Courses
* = Clinical Course

	Junior			Senior	
Concepts	Fall Courses	CR	Concepts	Fall Courses	CR
Illness across the lifespan	Pharmacology	3	Maximize health across lifespan	Case Management	2
	Technologies in Nursing	3		• *Collaboration*	
	• *Self-directed learning modules (use of NAPs) coordinated with Illness I.*			• *Population-based health care*	
	• *Front-loaded with the use of assistive technologies, e.g., SimMan*			Nursing Research	3
	• *Basic to advanced*			**General Elective or Creative Arts Core**	3
	Applied Pathophysiology I	3		Collaborative Care and Systems Thinking	4
	(taught by the SON)			• *Synthesis course*	
	• *Developmental patho. (e.g., diabetes across the lifespan, i.e., gestational, Type 1 and 2, MODY, systemic complications of DM)*			• *Case study format*	
				• *Chronic illness models*	
				• *Chronic multisystem management*	
				—Vertically integrated, wrap-around services)	
	Nursing Care of the Patient Experiencing Illness I	3		• *Effects of illness and hospitalization of the individual on the family and community*	
	• *Case study format*				
	• *Acute illness/acute exacerbations of chronic illness*			• *Nurse as the coordinator of care*	
	• *Systems failure*			• *Economic and reimbursement issues*	
	• *Pediatric disorders*				
	• *Obstetrical emergencies*			*Synergy in Nursing Practice: Management of Chronic Illness Across the Lifespan (community = 2 credits)*	5
	Synergy In Nursing Practice: Illness Across the Lifespan I (community = 2 credits)	3+2			
	• *Acute care with integrated clinical competencies (acute care instructor together on the clinical unit with consultation with other specialists)*				
	• *Evidence-based practice applications*				
		17			17

	Freshmen			Sophomores	
Concepts	**Spring Courses**	**CR**	**Concepts**	**Spring Courses**	**CR**
Professional socialization Professional ontology (assignments within these first level courses will include community involvement)	Ways of Knowing in Nursing • *Critical thinking* • *Scientific method/logic* • *Intro to nursing process and theory* • *Evidence-based practice* • *Teaching/learning process* • *Concept mapping* • *Cognitive/psychomotor/ affective learning* • *Use of technology* • *Self-esteem*	3	Science and art of health Mind-body interplay	A & P II	4
				Introductory Microbiology (BIOL 203/204)	4
				Health Assessment of Individuals and Community • *Adult* • *Older adult* • *Child* • *Pregnant woman* • *Community*	4

	Concepts of Professional Nursing Practice
	 • *Synergy Model*
	 • *History of nursing*
	 • *Intro to professional nsg*
	   —advocacy, agency, safety, quality, ethics, caring, legal, collaboration
	 • *Licensure*
	 • *Nursing roles*
	 • *Nursing organizations*
		3		Health Promotion
				 • *Health risk assessment/ behaviors*
				   —developmentally based (asthma, depression, home assessment, safety and violence, obesity
				 • *Cultural variations*
				 • *Health disparities*
				 • *Defense mechanisms*
				 • *Stress and anxiety*
				 • *Coping strategies*
				 • *Crisis intervention*
				 • *Threats to health in a community*
				 • *Ethical and legal issues*
					2

	Service Learning Strategies • *Service learning criteria*	1			
	Imaginative Literature	3		*Synergy in Nursing Practice: Healthy People II* • *Community/project-based* • *Normal assessment* • *Schools, homes* • *Evidence-based practice applications*	
	Transcultural Responses to Diversity in Health Care	3			
	Shaping of the Modern World	3			
		16			16

Juniors			Seniors		
Concepts	Spring Courses	CR	Concepts	Spring Courses	CR
Illness across the lifespan (cont.)	Community Health Concepts • *Public health models* —*Primary/secondary/ tertiary prevention and planning* —*precede-proceed model* • *Epidemiology* • *Capacities of communities* • *Building relationships with communities* • *Community planning* • *Disaster planning* • *Bioterrorism*	3	Collaborative wellness – illness facilitation	**General Elective or Creative Arts Core**	3
				Role Preparation/ NCLEX	1
	Applied Pathophysiology II • *Continuation of AP I* • *Include psychopathology*	3		Professional Concepts and Issues • *Synthesis/case study approach* • *Nursing policy* • *Law* • *Ethics* • *Professionalism*	3
	Fundamentals of Statistics	3		*Synergy in Nursing Practice (community = 2 credits) • *Capstone clinical course*	5+2
	Nursing Care of the Patient Experiencing Illness II • *Case study format* • *Acute multisystem failure including psychosocial care*	3			
	*Synergy In Nursing Practice: Illness Across the Lifespan II (community = 2 credits) • *Acute care/critical care with integrated clinical competencies* • *Acute care/community mental health* • *Evidence-based practice applications*	3+2			
		17			**14**

As the faculty became more comfortable with this model, we began to see how this model could also be used to reflect the combination of factors. For example, the Synergy Model is predicated on the premise that patient outcomes are enhanced when the nurses' competencies are compatible with the characteristics or needs of the patient. When applied in the educational system, that premise translates in that student learning outcomes are improved when faculty competencies are aligned with the learning needs of the students. Just as there are three spheres of influence in the practice model—the patient, the nurse, the system—so there are three spheres of influence on learning outcomes: the student (motivation, talent, inquisitiveness, basic abilities), the faculty (competence as teachers and as clinicians), and the system (university resources, clinical access, the curriculum). Figure 11.2 summarizes these variables within the spheres of the Synergy Model.

The Synergy Model for Nursing Education

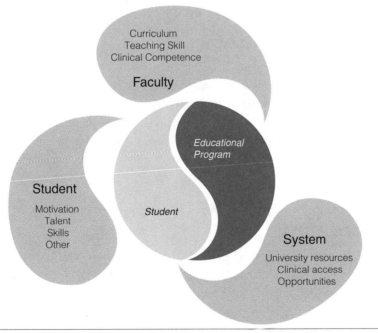

Figure 11.2.   The Synergy Model in Nursing Education.
Adapted with permission. (Curley, 1998).

Characteristics of Patients

While the examination of the characteristics of patients was scrutinized during this time, the role of these dimensions in the curriculum development was difficult to define. We looked at the possibility of having some "synergy" within the curriculum in pairing student level of achievement of nurse competency with some levels of patient characteristics. The outcome of that analysis was a general agreement that the nature of patient needs was too interrelated to attempt to divide between courses. We also feared that in emphasizing one patient characteristic over another, we ran the risk of fragmenting patients, or at least minimizing the importance of holistic approaches to patient care.

That was a few years ago. Since that time we have developed a stronger sense of the ways in which the needs of the patients guide student learning experiences. In the sophomore year of study, the patients tend to have more resources, are more open to learning, and have a greater capacity to participate in their care. In the junior year, where the focus is more on the acutely ill patients and their families, the full range of resources of the patient is challenged, as are the families' abilities to compensate. In that context the use of patient characteristics is more entwined with the overall evaluation of student learning.

Evaluation of Learning

The Synergy Model is also fully used by the students as they engage in self-evaluation practices. The overall theme of the curriculum clearly documents what students should be responsible for and the level of learning that they should have achieved. Furthermore, since all of the academic programming in the school uses the same basic framework, there is good communication and idea sharing between and among the various elements of the faculty.

The Synergy Model in Undergraduate and Graduate Education

In rethinking our academic approaches to the model, it is interesting to note the difference between the uses of the model in the graduate program and the undergraduate program. In the context of master's education for the specialist, it is clear that the emphasis is on the nurse's role in the various spheres of influence. In all the clinical specialties at the master's level, the role of the nurse with the patient is pivotal. However, in various specialties, the focus on the other spheres is variable. For example, the school has a large and highly successful forensic nursing option at the master's level. In this specialty area, the forensic nurse must collaborate and interact with staff nurses in emergency departments and other settings where crime victims turn for care. Here the forensic expert has considerable work to do to guide the practice of the emergency room nurse, who may not be an expert in sexual abuse or violent trauma. Therefore, in this specialty there is a high level of mentoring and collaboration between the forensic nurse and the staff nurse (nurse–nurse). Finally, since the victim, and perhaps the perpetrator, may move into other highly complex systems, in addition to the health-care arena, it is necessary that the forensic nurse be able to guide them through these systems. Similar comparisons could be made of nurses at the advanced level in other specialties.

In the undergraduate program, primary attention and concern is in the development of the nurse characteristics that foster quality patient care outcomes. While the graduate program entails the development of skill in each of the competency areas, there is more concern about applying those competencies within the broader framework of the health-care system. Although many of the support courses in the undergraduate program seek to develop within the student a broad perspective of the needs of the patient as a holistic entity—whether conceptualized as an individual, family, group, or community—there is substantially less attention to the larger context of health-care delivery in this program than in the master's.

In sum, the faculty at Duquesne University School of Nursing has found the Synergy Model to be an effective and meaningful framework for the organization of the undergraduate and master's programs. We are grateful for the work done by critical care nurses in developing a model that has such broad application in the academic setting and that can pave the way for the kind of "synergy" that needs to be fostered between the clinical and the educational setting.

The Synergy Model in Nursing Staff Development

JoAnn Grif Alspach, RN, MSN, EdD, FAAN

Since its developmental inception more than a decade ago, the AACN Synergy Model for Patient Care™ has represented an enlightened engagement in establishing not only theoretical, but actual linkage between clinical nursing practice and patient outcomes (Curley, 1996). The pivotal concept of this model portrays a patient-centered health-care system where patient and family needs dictate the competencies nurses must have to meet those needs (Edwards, 1999). Optimal patient care (quantifiable as patient outcomes) may then be achieved when synergy exists between patient needs and nurse competencies. This trio of interacting elements among the health-care system, the patient, and the nurse can be viewed holistically to highlight their mutual relationships (Curley, 1998).

One of the strengths of the Synergy Model is that it weaves the threads of patient needs into the nurse competencies necessary to meet those needs as a theoretical fabric. The model applies an evidence-based backing derived from and validated by bedside nurses that identifies the specific sets of patient and nurse characteristics most salient to effecting the synergy sought in patient care (Muenzen, Greenberg, & Pirrol, 2004). Patient and nurse characteristics, moreover, are portrayed not as static attributes or absolutes, but as human conditions that are variable in nature and degree. Although optimal patient outcomes require that the nurse be competent in all eight nurse dimensions, individual patients and their specific changing clinical situations will influence which nurse competencies are most important at any particular time. Just as each category of patient needs exists somewhere within a range of possible scenarios, each of the nurse competencies is also viewed along a continuum.

Following its initial dissemination to the nursing community, the Synergy Model has gradually gained increasingly wider audiences of nurses who acknowledge not only the relevance of its message, but the elegance of its vision. In 2005, a workshop for preceptor development served as the venue for introducing the notion that the Synergy Model could also be applied to the orientation component of nursing staff development (Alspach, 2005). The central thesis of this application was characterized in the following paired corollary, just as in the Synergy Model:

Optimal patient outcome can best be achieved when the *patient's characteristics* (expressed as need) are *matched* by the *nurse's characteristics* (expressed as competencies— see Figure 12.1).

The corollary holds true for a proposed Synergy Model for Orientation via Preceptorship—that *optimal orientation* of new nursing staff can best be achieved when the *orientee's characteristics* (expressed as needs) are *matched* by the *preceptor's characteristics* (expressed as competencies—see Figure 12.2).

In 2006, this fundamental assertion regarding the relevance and transferability of the Synergy Model to the orientation of new staff was extended to consider whether that supposition maintained continuity and consistency when subjected to the same set of assumptions that underlie the model (Muenzen et al., 2004). Alspach (2006) linked the nine assumptions guiding the Synergy Model to a corollary set of assumptions guiding the proposed Synergy Model for Preceptorship (see Table 12.1). No conceptual or practical issues were apparent in proposing these linkages, and no refutations were offered by those who responded to the solicitation for critique of the suggested linkages.

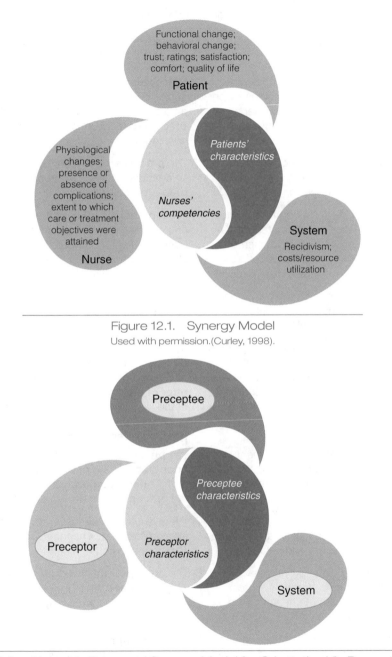

Figure 12.1.   Synergy Model
Used with permission.(Curley, 1998).

Figure 12.2.   Alspach's Proposed Synergy Model for Orientation Via Preceptorship
Used with permission. Alspach, J.G. Preceptor Empowerment #101 and #102.
Mastery Session presented at 2005 AACN National Institute, New Orleans, LA, May 2005.
Adapted with permission. (Curley, 1998).

Table 12.1. Assumptions Guiding Synergy Model Applications.

AACN Synergy Model for Patient Care	Alspach's Proposed Synergy Model for Preceptorship
1) **Patients** are biological, psychological, social, and spiritual entities who present at a particular developmental stage. The whole **patient** (body, mind, and spirit) must be considered.	1) **Preceptees*** are biological, psychological, social, and spiritual entities who present at a particular developmental stage. The whole **preceptee** (body, mind, and spirit) must be considered.
2) The **patient, family,** and **community** all contribute to providing a context for the **nurse-patient** relationship.	2) The **preceptee** and community contribute to providing a context for the **preceptor-preceptee** relationship.
3) **Patients** can be described by a number of characteristics. All characteristics are connected and contribute to each other. Characteristics cannot be looked at in isolation.	3) **Preceptees** can be described by a number of characteristics. All characteristics are connected and contribute to each other. Characteristics cannot be looked at in isolation.
4) Similarly, nurses can be described on a number of **dimensions**. The interrelated dimensions paint a profile of the **nurse.**	4) Similarly, **preceptors** can be described on a number of dimensions. The interrelated dimensions paint a profile of the **preceptor.**
5) A goal of **nursing** is to **restore** a **patient** to an optimal level of **wellness** as defined by the **patient. Death** can be an acceptable outcome, in which the goal of **nursing** care is to move a **patient** toward a peaceful **death.**	5) A goal of **orientation** is to ensure the **preceptee demonstrates** an optimal level of **competency** as defined by the **hospital. Rescinding an offer of employment** can be an acceptable outcome, in which the goal of **preceptorship** is to move **preceptee** toward an **alternative position or employer.**
6) The **nurse** creates the environment for the care of the **patient.** The environment of care also affects what the **nurse** can do.	6) The **preceptor** creates the environment for the **orientation** of the **preceptee.** The environment of the **orientation program** also affects what the **preceptor** can do.
7) There is interrelatedness between impact areas, which may change as the experience, situation, and setting change.	7) There is interrelatedness between impact areas, which may change as the experience, situation, and setting change.
8) The **nurse** may work to optimize outcomes for **patients, families,** health-care providers, and the health-care system.	8) The **preceptor** may work to optimize outcomes for **preceptees,** health-care providers, the work unit, and the health-care system.
9) The **nurse** brings his or her background to each situation, including various levels of education/knowledge and skills/experience.	9) The **preceptor** brings his or her background to each situation, including various levels of education/knowledge and skills/experience.

Used with permission. Alspach, J.G. (2006). Extending the Synergy Model to preceptorship: A preliminary proposal. Critical Care Nurse. 26(2), 10-13.

*Preceptee is synonymous with orientee—a newly hired member of the staff.

This chapter will further the proposal that the Synergy Model can be readily applied to not only the relationship between a preceptor and orientee during the orientation program, but how this framework can be used to realign all major elements of staff development, to sharpen the specific focus of staff orientation programs, and to describe how the preceptor's role and preceptor development programs would be modified by this integration. As a prelude to that discussion, some background related to terms and traditional approaches to relevant aspects of staff development are needed.

Staff Development

The American Nurses Association (ANA) defines nursing *professional development* as "the lifelong process of active participation by nurses in learning activities that assist in developing and maintaining their continuing competence, enhance their professional practice, and support achievement of their career goals" (ANA, 2000, p. 4). The activities encompassed by nursing professional development include the three potentially overlapping domains of academic education, staff development, and continuing education. In contrast to undertaking academic courses toward completing a degree or other academic program or pursuing any form of systematic learning that might enrich a nurse's general knowledge, attitudes, or skills, the term *staff development* refers more specifically to employer-sponsored and/or provided educational programs related to the work setting. These activities comprise orientation, in-service education, and continuing education programs (ANA, 2000).

Orientation introduces new staff to the culture, philosophy, goals, policies, role expectations, and other elements required for functioning effectively in a particular work setting; verifies the competency of newly hired staff to function in their assigned role, on their assigned work setting; and assists in socializing new staff into the workplace. *In-service education* assists nurses in maintaining and continuing to develop their job-related competence throughout the duration of their employment and, within staff development, *continuing education* affords learning that may enrich any nurse's professional career (ANA, 2000).

Reconceptualizing the Purpose of Staff Development Programs

If synergy is to be achieved between the patient and the nurse providing care for that patient, then the nurse-patient relationship must remain the focal point not only for nurses who provide direct patient care, but for those who practice nursing in complementary spheres of professional responsibility such as staff development, management, administration, or research. Within this patient-centered context, then, application and integration of a Synergy Model framework into nursing staff development would affect the following:

- The primary purpose of orientation would no longer culminate in socializing new staff, familiarizing them with the nuances of their new employer, or even with verifying their competence to do the jobs for which they have just been hired. Rather, the primary purpose of orientation within the Synergy Model would incorporate and extend beyond these traditional outcomes to capture the patient as well. Within the Synergy Model, then, the primary purpose of orientation is verifying that the newly hired nurse actually provides nursing care that meets the behavioral criteria included at Level 1 of the nurse competencies (see Figure 12.3). The focal point for orientation thereby shifts from the nurse to the nurse-patient interactions that represent those of a nurse at the competent level (Level 1) of nursing practice.

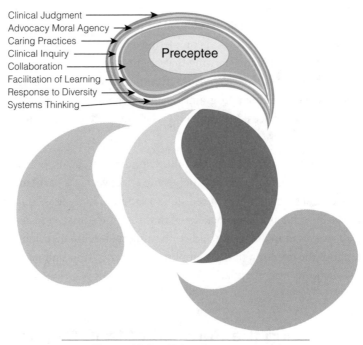

Figure 12.3. Primary purpose of orientation within the Synergy Model.

- The primary purpose of in-service education would lengthen its focus commensurately, shifting its emphasis from not only assisting nurses in maintaining and enhancing their job-related competence, but extending these concerns to furthering the nurse's professional development from Level 1 through Levels 2 and 3 along the practice continuum for each nurse competency identified as essential to providing optimal patient care.

- The primary purpose of continuing education would, in kind, advance beyond forms of organized learning that augment the nurse's professional career to learning that enhances any of the nurse competency areas that contribute to provision of optimal patient care.

Before leaving these points, it is important to clarify that the changes in staff development that evolve from its integration into a Synergy Model approach to patient care neither suggest nor imply that the traditional focus of staff development on augmentation of the nurse's knowledge, attitudes, and skills is in any way erroneous, deficient, or misdirected. To the contrary, optimizing the competence that the nurse brings to every patient care situation is precisely the objective desired. The enlightenment on this issue owing to the Synergy Model framework is its illumination of two considerations that might otherwise be overlooked:

1. Unless nurses actually evidence the enhanced capabilities afforded through staff development programs in their interactions with patients, such learning will not contribute to optimal patient care and no synergistic effect will be forthcoming;

2. Although a multitude of nurse competency areas might be enhanced by staff development and thereby improve the quality of patient care, to date only eight have been systematically and scientifically verified to do so. Unless one or more of those nurse competency areas is augmented, there is little evidence to suggest that the synergy sought between nurse and patient will be realized.

Sharpening the Focus of Orientation

With the Synergy Model now extending the reach of orientation to embrace the nature and quality of the nurse-patient relationship in all competency areas identified as relevant, a number of other facets related to the orientation process will require refocusing in order for the targeted end-point of synergy to be reached. Some of the manifestations of this improved visual acuity for orientation could include the following:

Within the Synergy Model, then, the primary purpose of orientation is verifying that the newly hired nurse actually provides nursing care to patients that meet all of the behavioral criteria included at Level 1 of the nurse competencies. The focal point for orientation thereby shifts from the nurse to the nurse-patient interactions that represent those of a nurse at the competent level (Level 1) of nursing practice.

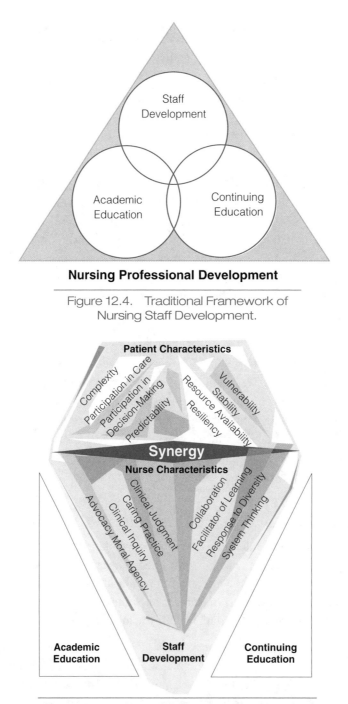

Nursing Professional Development

Figure 12.4.   Traditional Framework of
Nursing Staff Development.

Figure 12.5.   Alspach's Framework of Nursing
Staff Development Within the Synergy Model.
© 2007 JoAnn Grif Alspach

- Reconstructing the traditional organizational framework for nursing staff development (see Figure 12.4) to one more consistent with the Synergy Model. A preliminary example of a framework for nursing staff development within the Synergy Model is suggested in Figure 12.5.

- Operationally relocating traditional components of the orientation process into the reconstructed framework, for example.

- Traditional emphasis on assessment and verification of the nurse orientee's clinical competency and validation that his or her direct patient care is consistent with facility policies and procedures—as well as with accrediting, regulatory, and statutory requirements and related imperatives—could be largely relocated under the nurse characteristic of clinical judgment.

  - Traditional requirements not related to direct patient care, such as fire and electrical safety, response to natural or man-made disasters, or chemical or biological incidents, can be located within whichever competency area is most fitting, for example, collaboration, systems thinking, and so on.

  - Traditional emphasis on socializing new staff into the workplace could be relocated under the nurse characteristic of collaboration and/or response to diversity.

  - Traditional emphasis on introducing new staff to the culture, philosophy, goals, role expectations, and other elements unique to a particular work setting may be relocated to whichever nurse characteristic they most suitably fit, for example, systems thinking, advocacy/moral agency, response to diversity, and the like.

- Providing any necessary instructional support in Synergy Model elements to all nurse orientees, for example.

  - An introduction to the Synergy Model with description of its implications and adoption at that facility.

  - Definition and explanation of the patient characteristics and their tri-level continuum along the health-illness spectrum.

  - Definition and explanation of the nurse characteristics and their tri-level continuum along the nursing practice spectrum.

  - Explanation of how the model is evidenced and experienced throughout orientation, inservice, and continuing education offerings, as well as in subsequent employment issues such as performance appraisals and clinical advancement procedures at that facility.

- Adding any neglected Synergy Model elements to appraisal segments of the orientation program, for example.
  - Ensuring that orientee assessments and evaluation procedures include all nurse competency areas.
  - Ensuring that completion of orientation requires all staff nurse orientees to demonstrate all behavioral criteria listed at nursing practice Level 1 (Competent) for all nurse competencies.
- Providing any necessary instructional support in Synergy Model elements to all nurse orientees, for example.
  - An introduction to the Synergy Model with description of its implications and adoption at that facility.
- Curriculum design, content distributions, and time allocations for the orientation program might also be influenced by the same research originally targeted for determining content distribution in the AACN Certification Corporation's CCRN certification exam. Since the most recent survey of nursing practice in critical care determined that the great majority of critical care nursing time is expended in activities related to the Clinical Judgment competency area, 80% of content in the CCRN examination is targeted to that area, with the remaining 20% distributed among the remaining seven nurse competencies. Although the composition and circumstances of nurse orientees at a given facility would surely affect those allocations, the relative importance of various content areas gleaned from the Synergy Model would afford nurse educators with a good starting point for decision-making related to the relative proportion of instructional and evaluation times during the orientation program that should be planned for each of the various nurse competency areas.
- The evaluation tools (e.g., checklists or comparable means) used for documentation of an orientee's progress in completing orientation would also need revision to ensure that these devices reflected not merely a long enumeration of the new hire's knowledge, attitudes, and skills. Since orientation using the Synergy Model encompasses the nurse's actual interactions with the patient, then "successful completion" of orientation requires that the newly hired nurse demonstrate patient care consistent with all of the behavioral criteria included at Level 1 of the nurse competencies.

Synergy Integration Into the Preceptor's Role

Preceptors have two primary spheres of responsibility: orientation and integration of new staff (Alspach, 2000).

1) *Orientation*—Preceptors are responsible for assisting the newly hired nurse in completing the orientation process for his or her designated position as well as to the assigned patient care unit, including both the unit's physical features as well as its formal policies, procedures, and operations.

2) *Integration*—Preceptors are responsible for facilitating the professional and social integration of new staff members with their colleagues and coworkers, and with familiarizing them with the formal and informal culture and mores of the work setting.

In fulfilling these responsibilities, preceptors serve in three primary roles (Alspach, 2000; see Figure 12.6):

Preceptor Roles

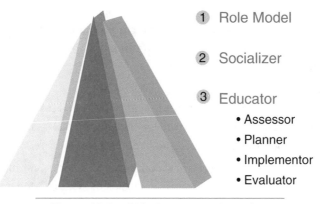

1 Role Model

2 Socializer

3 Educator
- Assessor
- Planner
- Implementor
- Evaluator

Figure 12.6. Primary preceptor roles.

© 2005 JoAnn Grif Alspach. Adapted from: Alspach, Grif. Preceptor Empowerment #101 and #102. Mastery Session presented at 2005 AACN National Teaching Institute, New Orleans, LA; May 2005.

1) **Role model:** wherein the preceptor personally exemplifies how the orientee is expected to carry out the duties associated with his or her designated position in the assigned work setting.

2) **Socializer**: wherein the preceptor welcomes and facilitates the new staff member's integration with peers, coworkers, and employer.

3) **Educator:** wherein the preceptor provides instructional support to the orientee by enacting any or all of the following subroles:

> *Assessor* of orientee's learning needs related to orientation outcomes
>
> *Planner* of learning experiences for the orientee
>
> *Implementer* of learning plans and activities
>
> *Evaluator* of the orientee's job performance

As changes are instituted in the orientation program, the preceptor's roles will necessarily need modification to accommodate the program changes. The most direct influences that enveloping orientation within a Synergy Model framework would likely impose on the preceptor's roles and responsibilities include:

- Reflection among current preceptors regarding how institution of a model of patient care based on the Synergy Model influences nursing practice at their facility (in general), on their patient unit (in particular), and in their orientation program for new staff (in detail).

- Rethinking their personal perspective on the role of a preceptor to enable shifting from the traditional emphasis on imparting information; teaching clinical procedures; demonstrating role execution; and validating the orientee's knowledge, attitudes, and skills to verifying that the orientee actually applies these capabilities in providing patient care on his or her assigned unit.

- Anticipating the need to provide considerable additional support to new graduates in making the transition from knowledge acquisition, task management, and skill mastery to transfer these elements into hands-on patient care.

- Ensuring that orientee appraisals and competency verification procedures include documentation of the orientee's performance of all Synergy Model nurse characteristics at least at the Competent (Level 1) performance for each.

- Providing, reinforcing, and augmenting any background instruction related to the Synergy Model patient and nurse characteristics that were not included in system- or facility-wide central staff orientation programs.

Synergy Integration Into Preceptor Development Programs

In addition to adding the above elements to the existing preceptor development program, adoption of a Synergy Model framework for nursing will likely require enhanced emphasis on two specific facets of those programs:

1. **Assessment and evaluation of orientees**—Health-care facilities will need to determine how they wish to restructure their orientation programs via the Synergy Model. In so doing, each facility will need to make decisions regarding the specific behavioral criteria they will employ for both appraising and evaluating new staff in each of the nurse characteristics. Many facilities will likely both incorporate the behavioral criteria already stipulated by AACN and add others to meet local, regional, or regulatory mandates. Although all facilities will have preexisting requirements of orientees for competency areas related to clinical judgment and facilitation of learning, many may currently lack comparable appraisal criteria for areas such as advocacy and moral agency, systems thinking, or clinical inquiry. The preceptor will need to use whatever criteria the facility determines for this purpose, so any issues or problems with clarity, ambiguity, interpretation, or documentation related to those criteria should be ironed out before the new preceptor actually begins working with new staff.

2. **Instruction**—For any new staff that need instructional support for meeting expectations related to the nurse competencies, prospective preceptors will need to know how to provide any necessary instruction in these areas. At some point in the future, academic nursing programs may well provide this foundation for student nurses, but until then, orientation programs and preceptors will need to provide any necessary supplementation. As a result, preceptors will need instruction not only on how to teach the more familiar aspects of clinical judgment such as critical thinking, but on how they can effectively and efficiently teach less familiar practice areas such as caring practices, advocacy, collaboration, clinical inquiry, and systems thinking.

Summary

As the Synergy Model continues to gain preeminence in clarifying the beneficial relationship between nursing practice and optimal patient outcomes, its applications to other nursing functions such as management, administration, staff development, and research become increasingly apparent and visible. This chapter describes a natural and seamless integration that can be achieved between the Synergy Model and nursing staff development that complements the former by transforming the latter into a consistent execution of nursing functions that maintains the primacy and quality of nurse-patient interactions as its centerpiece.

The Synergy Model: A Framework for Professional Development and Transformation

Chapter

13

Christine M. Pacini, PhD, RN

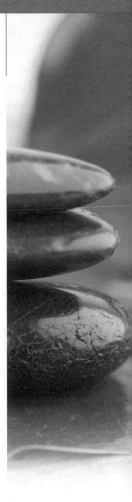

Introduction

Change in health care as a microcosm of the broader universe is occurring at a rate that makes it almost impossible to keep up. Mechanisms for delivering service, generating relevant products/ processes and reconfiguring systems are becoming increasingly complex. Seemingly some of the most formidable characteristics of these systems are that they are inherently uncontrollable and unpredictable, thereby requiring new models and approaches for responsive intervention. For example, concepts such as shared leadership, healing sanctuaries, servant leadership, communities of caring, and self-managed work teams are evolving in support of values related to patient/family centrality, customer-focused behavior, process improvement, lean thinking, safety, and high-quality clinical/behavioral outcomes.

One of the key problems is that past approaches to leading, managing, and learning are far less relevant in environments characterized by values associated with newer knowledge about how change occurs and how individuals think and behave (e.g.,

Goleman, 1998; Greenleaf, 1996; Porter-O'Grady & Malloch, 2003). In particular, traditional customs about teaching/learning with regard to aims, content, and methods may now serve as impediments to organizational growth and understanding of models of transformation. The content of transformation requires a movement away from industrial/linear thinking toward a focus on integration, outcomes, flexibility, responsiveness, holism, contingency thinking, and anticipatory openness to possibility.

The AACN Synergy Model for Patient Care™ provides a framework for nursing practice driven by the needs and characteristics of patients and the demands of the health-care environment *predicted for the future.* The fundamental premise of the model is that patient characteristics drive nurses' competencies. When patients' characteristics and nurses' competencies match and synergize, patients' outcomes will be optimized. This paradigm is extraordinarily relevant and elegant in that it assumes professional accountability and authority for a clearly articulated set of competencies that vary in light of *patient* requirements. Moreover, those competencies represent contemporary nursing practice and reflect a dynamic integration of wisdom, experience, values, and knowledge. As such, the model provides a compelling perspective when compared with prior approaches that didn't adequately account for the ever-increasing complexities manifested by patients in contexts marked by variability and unpredictability.

Transformational Clinical Education

As health-care and nursing organizations mobilize to design and implement products and processes that demonstrate relevance to the principles and assumptions noted above, it is apparent that there exists a growing dissonance between what is required in the clinical world and what is incorporated in educational programming. From the perspective of academic nursing, it has been my experience that curricular relevance and integrity are only enhanced when faculty and clinical nursing leaders (e.g., administrators, managers, clinical educators, advanced practice nurses) engage in mutual, ongoing, regularly scheduled, honest, participative dialogue/discourse about evolving realities and operational standards/phenomena in practice. In a fully realized, mutual partnership, this dialogue rests within legitimate venues of authority and governance. That is, clinical representatives routinely participate in established academic committee venues. Conversely, academic faculty must necessarily partner and participate in similar clinical governance structures. In addition, new partnership models that proactively and substantively link clinical instruction activities with actual practice and team membership/participation are essential for transforming student development from distanced/simulated instructional activity to fully engaged learning.

New paradigms of change should influence processes that impede or delay opportunities for innovation. It is imperative that creativity, knowledge utilization, responsiveness, and openness prevail as normative behavior and expectations in the "new age." As benchmarking related to expected *outcomes* of clinical performance is the industry standard for measuring organizational value, so must we apply similar constructs of expected, predictable, reliable, measurable outcomes with respect to educational productivity. Organizations, whose means of survival and growth depend on high quality clinical practice that is tailored and responsive to customers' needs and expectations, are increasingly taking on greater responsibility for workforce development. In addition, there is substantive variability in quality and performance of entry-level graduates. Thus, it behooves us to carefully engage in the examination of educational outcomes from a perspective that represents the best thinking of both academic faculty and clinical practitioners.

Even assuming that greater educational synergy will be accomplished in the near term by implementing enhanced opportunities for interactive dialogue and instructional redesign between academic and clinical partners, there will always remain the requirement for ongoing educational intervention in our practice settings. First and foremost, the transition from an academic setting to the practice arena is monumental. Pace, volume, and acuity provide the context for new learning and application of principles in real time. Complexity and variability in processes, environment, and personnel further complicate one's trajectory for learning, whether one is new to the profession or new to the organization. Unreasonable expectations for contribution and productivity may add to the "mixture" of risk and insecurity. Growing realization that one has actual authority for a defined scope of practice and is accountable for patient outcomes can provoke a sense of personal distress about limited capacity or evoke a crisis of trust about others and their level of competency or support. In any instance, the implications for learning and development are as complex, variable, and/or demanding as are the prevailing context and related content.

From the perspective of clinical nursing practice, it is my experience that common implications for educational programming are characterized by the need for breadth, depth, continuity, responsiveness, regulatory sensibility, flexibility, 24/7 availability, just-in-time requirements, etc. More importantly, the utilization of a conceptual model to provide infrastructure that decreases variability among nurses in any functional capacity is central to set a firm direction about where an enterprise needs to go (Kerfoot, Lavandero, Cox, Triola, Pacini, & Hanson, 2006).

Whether one engages in direct patient care, serves in a management role, educates staff, participates in the work of inquiry, and so on, the motivation for productivity and evaluation of success is driven by the understanding of patient-nurse centrality as embodied in the Synergy Model. Tenets of the model further assume and prescribe that performance and role expectations of nurses practicing therein are living a *professional* reality. That is, behavioral characteristics embodying clinical judgment (incorporating things such as wisdom, reasoning, intellectual capacity, innovation, and so on), advocacy/moral agency, caring practice, collaboration, responsiveness to diversity (broadly defined), facilitation of learning, and systems thinking reflect a cadre of competencies essential to meeting patient needs. These are not the tenets of ritualistic, task-focused practice. Furthermore, patient characteristics are identified and reflect an *integration* about manifestations that necessarily drive/predicate a professional response. Characteristics of vulnerability, resiliency, stability, complexity, predictability, and so on are not routinely managed from a stimulus-response perspective, nor are they adequately addressed by providers practicing within a hierarchical, maternalistic/paternalistic scheme of intervention. Rather, the underlying assumption is that patients/families are not bystanders or passive recipients of one-size-fits-all care—they are actively engaged participants in care and decision-making.

Further study and analysis of the model reveal opportunities and options for revolutionizing conventional approaches to education in clinical settings. Current practice often focuses on accomplishing regulatory mandates/requirements that may serve to justify the utilization of methods that have very little to do with professional development. Indeed, practice reality requires intervention, documentation, and validation of certain mandates, but is that all there is? In a clinical environment shaped by Synergy, that certainly is *not* all there is. Synergy is prescriptive for an approach that moves beyond requirement to possibility.

With Synergy, it is no longer acceptable to view a group of newly hired RNs as a collection of people conveniently clustered together for the purpose of "giving them what they need." Nurses manifest different strengths and needs with respect to each of the characteristics. Thus, models of learning needs assessment need to be reconfigured in light of nurse attributes conceptualized on a continuum (vs. a dichotomous interpretation of competence). Integration of the concept of safe passage (Curley, 1998) necessarily implies that the trajectory of orientation, learning, and ongoing development must be shaped by the reality of patient-focused phenomena and outcomes. Differentiated practice and support of professional development require ongoing competency-based educational programming that facilitates skill development characterized by judgment, intellect, and contribution. Transformational learning experiences require approaches and methods beyond traditional means of lecture and demonstration. Experiential learning occurring under the guidance of well-prepared clinical coaches or preceptors will facilitate the development of proficiency and expertise.

Application of the Synergy Model to Clinical Nursing Education

The journey to educational reformation and transformation can be unequivocally shaped by the Synergy Model. Assumptions about key elements of educational processes and products should necessarily parallel constructs embedded in the model. For example, job documents of clinical educators and education specialists can be configured in terms of the nurse characteristics. Behaviors and criteria for performance evaluation should be described in terms of clinical judgment, clinical inquiry, caring practices, etc. For example, the work of clinical judgment as manifested by an education specialist would incorporate high level intellectual expectations around the processes associated with teaching/learning:

> Demonstrate excellence in educational practice through systematic assessment of learning needs of clinical and educational staff, analysis of data/evidence, prioritized planning in accordance with strategic directives, curricular design congruent with current and projected benchmarks of excellence, implementation of instructional methods consistent with broad organizational requirements and learner needs, and evaluation of outcomes in terms of contribution to organizational aims, vision and directives.

The characteristic of clinical inquiry demands that an education specialist would:

> Incorporate pertinent nursing, patient care, and/or educational research into staff development programs and materials; conduct evaluation research to determine the effectiveness of educational programs to meet desired clinical, service, people, and fiscal outcomes; analyze and evaluate educational structures, processes, and outcomes in accordance with national standards and benchmarks and implement change processes that positively impact expected outcomes; apply performance improvement methods to continuously enhance programmatic impact and contribution to strategic aims; mentor staff in the use and application of valid and reliable methods to evaluate competency and performance.

These are but two examples of how educator job expectations can be delineated using the nurse characteristics of the Synergy Model as an organizing framework.

In addition, it is critical that practice be differentiated between master's-prepared specialists and clinical educators. Expectations related to leadership and expertise in assessment, curricular design, program management, outcomes analysis, and testing/

measurement/evaluation must be incorporated in the specialists' job document. Education specialists should also be charged with ongoing development and coaching of clinical educators in the application of standards of practice for nursing professional development. They would serve as "master teachers." Non-master's-prepared clinical educators generally manifest extraordinary readiness and competence in *implementation* of educational products and processes at a grass-roots level. Furthermore, assessment of clinical educators' performance must necessarily be defined in terms of safe passage. That is, the trajectory of learning within the time frame of orientation is conceptualized as a highly interactive partnership among the orientee, the preceptor, and the clinical manager. Charged with oversight of these triads, the clinical educator must intervene with one, or any, or all of the participants to guarantee a safe passage for healthy learning during this critical period.

Patient characteristics can also serve as operational descriptors for learners. As educators, we should take the position that learners vary across the same dimensions as patients. Thus, mechanisms for assessing learning needs could be reconfigured in recognition of the fact that resiliency, vulnerability, complexity, etc., are detectable manifestations for all kinds of recipients of nursing intervention, including nursing orientees and others engaged in programs of learning. It is also hypothesized that utilization of "ranking" on a continuum (vs. dichotomous assessment of task accomplishment) will provide more useful baseline data for ongoing developmental planning.

Orientation

Traditional models of orientation customarily provide newly hired employees with a substantial volume of required information early on. Variations on this theme have incorporated Web-based/online validation options, self-study programs, and other approaches for orienting individuals to a wide variety of regulatory/mandatory requirements. It has been my observation over many years and across several organizations that a common view is that we have a captive audience of learners and a lot of information to "give" them, so let's plow through it all and get it "over with." I can't begin to recall how many times I've heard the suggestion: "Well, we can add that to orientation when we've got them all together." Any clinical educator or preceptor can easily describe the glassy-eyed look of orientees after a week of being on the receiving end of content saturation and high-volume skill/competency validation.

Clearly there is evidence in the literature that many organizations are applying new approaches, content, and methods for evaluating orientees and outcomes of these important programs. The concern is that we are approaching a level of hypervigilance when it comes to issues of regulatory compliance and mandatory education. Progression toward clinical transformation and fully realized professional practice will not occur if educational resources are stacked so predominantly toward accomplishing these limited, though essential, aims. Critical distinctions need to occur in curriculum design from the outset. For example, tenets of educational theory combined with standards for professional development would necessarily limit early orientation content and methods around a focus of what is essential and necessary to know. Attention to patient safety, cue recognition representing impending crisis and need for support, and resource availability (e.g., delegating up to supportive/knowledgeable colleagues) provides direction for inclusion and exclusion of relevant content. The implementation of orientation should be a temporally organized experience with provision for coordinated/planned interface between didactic and clinical instruction. Mutuality and learners' needs must drive teacher interventions. When there is synergistic interaction, learning outcomes will be enhanced. It is also essential that we begin to substantively adopt the "commandment" that orientation does *not* conclude on the day that an individual is "counted into staffing." Current economic models that drive orientation have obliterated most sensibility about assuming a developmental posture in our relationships with new employees. It seems that if someone doesn't "hit the ground running" at the conclusion of some arbitrary time frame, the inference is that there is something wrong with the individual—notwithstanding the likelihood that we have assigned the new employee to an off-shift with limited resources related to educational or developmental support. Having said that, and clearly understanding that there is a requirement for fiscal responsibility, the notion of orientation redesign should take into account the need for dedicated, periodic interventions that will continuously facilitate professional growth and development in our settings. This position is derived from and substantiated by the work of Benner and her colleagues (Benner, 1984; Benner, Hooper-Kyriakidis, & Stannard, 1999; Benner, Tanner, & Chesla, 1996) who have so clearly documented the trajectory of skill and knowledge acquisition for nursing.

The Synergy Model provides an infrastructure that has a high degree of utility for orientation redesign. For example, by using the constructs of safety and safe passage, early orientation, weeks 1-4, would be dedicated to accomplishing those essential competencies and tasks that preserve the safety of patients and prepare the nurse to function within the context of a new setting. As nurses have accumulated some operational experience in their new setting or role, the next phase of orientation, weeks 5-12, should provide individuals with opportunities to debrief and develop their practice around principles embedded in the patient side of the Synergy Model. The overall aim would be to support nurses as they apply and utilize the model in practice, especially as it relates to patient/family manifestations of the characteristics. A conscious shift in focus, away from task and procedure, toward seeing the nuances of the patient/family through the lens of resiliency, vulnerability, stability, complexity, etc., facilitates the development of a lived practice that is patient-centric in essence. A third phase of orientation, week 12 or thereafter, would provide individuals with an opportunity to come to understand the opportunities for professional development or advancement within their organization. The aim would be to provide nursing staff with useful and appropriate developmental tools to accomplish performance expectations and achieve professional success. The nurse side of the model would provide the organizing framework for this phase of orientation.

Professional Development

The American Nurses Association (2000) has outlined the scope and standards of practice for nursing professional development. Several philosophical statements direct one to interpret that the creative work of professional development requires a substantive commitment far beyond obligations associated with meeting regulatory or task-focused requirements. The work of facilitating the development of fully engaged nursing professionals transcends a notion of something "nice to do" to something essential and necessary to do. In addition and as noted previously, the acquisition of skill and knowledge in a clinical practice setting as described by Benner and her colleagues (Benner, 1984; Benner, Tanner et al., 1996; Benner, Hooper-Kyriakidis et al., 1999) requires ongoing developmental intervention as one progresses through the stages of early practice, competency, proficiency, and expertise. Again, the Synergy Model provides an exemplary framework for designing and implementing a comprehensive educational approach to support the progression and advancement of nurses in an environment that recognizes and rewards differentiated practice and clinical leadership.

Using the eight nurse characteristics (i.e., clinical judgment, clinical inquiry, caring practices, response to diversity, advocacy/moral agency, facilitation of learning, collaboration, systems thinking), one can conceptualize and construct an educational program that integrates knowledge development that can only be acquired by being in the presence of patients and families and that which can be enhanced or facilitated using didactic methods.

If one considers the development of clinical judgment, caring practice, and advocacy/moral agency, for example, it is hard to think that skills such as those are honed in any type of artificial setting. Rather, a beginning nurse develops clinical wisdom and the skills of involvement, engagement, and advocacy by being present to patients/families while being guided and nurtured by other nurses who practice at a proficient or expert level. For example, advanced beginners live in a world of insecurity and concern about the adequacy of their performance overall. They can be assisted by offering opportunities to review and contemplate over situations that did not go particularly well. It is imperative that advanced beginners work in environments where they feel secure asking questions. In order to maintain a safe clinical experience for patients, it is essential that beginners' inexperience not be judged as personal inadequacy, but recognized as an expected phase in the development of clinical judgment. Most hazardous to patients are those environments that are interpersonally threatening, that punish early mistakes, or that set up barriers to the free exchange of questions from advanced beginners. Despite the reality that "official" orientation may conclude after 4, 6, 8, 10, or 12 weeks, it is crucial to sustain some type of coaching relationship for at least 6 months. Giles and Moran (1989) discovered that the option of maintaining a recognized relationship between each advanced beginner and one experienced nurse for the full duration was most efficacious.

The journey to competency, proficiency, and expertise around the aspects of judgment, caring practice, and advocacy also requires unique developmental opportunities. Benner et al. (1996) suggest that new kinds of staff development be implemented for nurses who are becoming proficient. Narratives of learning told in small groups that focus on changing one's perspectives and expectations in a clinical situation can be very instructive and support the advancement of skill development in problem identification and responsiveness to salient patient manifestations. It is important for the individual who leads this type of intervention to publicly sanction the learner's recognition of changing clinical relevance and legitimize the correlated thinking as being astute and flexible. This instructional stance is very different from criticizing the individual for having the incorrect perception or plan from the outset. Instead the developmental and instructional work is to flesh out the thinking and judgment exhibited by the nurse that ebbs and flows with evolving and changing clinical data.

Perhaps the most important consideration in facilitating learning with competent or proficient nurses is the reality that one's authentic engagement, support, acceptance, and receptivity can actually contribute to the individual's formation around moral agency. Benner, Tanner, and Chesla (1996) tell us that this is a very powerful obligation, and the work of assisting nurses in knowing what things can and cannot wait has substantive implications for the well-being of patients and families. In all, it is essential to recognize that professional development around the constructs of judgment, caring, and agency requires personal investment, coaching, and sophisticated, just-in-time interventions that occur in direct response to the manifestation of clinical phenomena as experienced by the learner. This is not the "stuff" of textbooks and classroom instruction. However, these skills will not be developed randomly either. Rather, models of ongoing clinical development using distinct instructional methods that occur in the lived experience of practice are required to evolve a cadre of nurses who demonstrate expertise around the critical characteristics of clinical judgment, caring practice, and agency.

When one considers the nurse characteristics associated with inquiry, response to diversity, facilitation of learning, collaboration, and systems thinking, it is conceivable to think that one could construct a developmental curriculum that enhances key skills associated with these domains of practice. The focus of this type of instruction would serve to facilitate the enhancement of competencies related to professional contribution and leadership at the unit level. In an informed and progressive nursing culture, concepts related to authentic professionalism, transformation, authority, and accountability for practice and clinical leadership would necessarily infuse the developmental program.

At Clarian Health Partners Inc., the Synergy curriculum was designed for registered nurses who elected to apply for promotion within the Clinical Advancement Program (CAP). The prevailing aim of this sequence of modules (courses) was to enhance the development of proficient practitioners who would assume positions of clinical leadership in the domain of clinical practice (versus management or education). This curriculum provides an example of a model whereby the Synergy nurse characteristics were used to organize a professional development program that extended beyond the confines of orientation and served to enhance the development of nurses in various stages of practice. By design, classes were offered during all shifts and on weekends, so that all nurses could elect to participate. Certain course elements and some of the modules had online options for completion. Managers were free to use the curriculum as a tool for individualized professional development and/or encouragement. Interactive methods, small class size, and utilization of the seminar format were incorporated to enhance opportunities for dialogue and active learning processes. Modules were configured as follows:

Enhancing Coaching and Effective Communication Skills in the Peer Review Process

- Differentiate among the concepts of precepting, mentoring, and coaching in regard to definition, purpose, characteristics, and scope
- Determine the skill set that one needs to be an effective coach for staff
- Identify a specific area within one's care environment in which one could effect change
- Compare and contrast effective and ineffective peer review situations
- Provide constructive feedback to peers to enhance their clinical practice regarding psychomotor, affective, and cognitive skills

Teamwork, Patient Safety, and Conflict Management

- Compare and contrast characteristics of groups that function as a team and those that do not
- Identify common problems with achieving the ideal of "team" and the effects on patient safety
- Identify common clinical situations that result in conflict between patient-nurse, family-nurse, nurse-physician, nurse-other health team member, peer-peer
- Describe methods to enhance conflict management skills

Engaging as a Clinical Leader

- Identify a variety of clinical tools for evaluating and guiding practice (e.g., algorithms, protocols, care maps, teaching records, etc.)
- Identify sources and/or resources of professional standards
- Apply quality improvement methodology to clinical practice outcomes
- Evaluate quality markers/data sources for determining unit population outcomes
- Extract practice implications to improve outcome achievement for population or unit-based trajectory of care
- Describe unit-based shared leadership (governance) structure(s) and identify opportunities for contribution
- Distinguish shared leadership (governance) from administration

Effecting Change in the Practice Environment: Unit as System

- Utilize elements/processes embedded within business planning and/or project management frameworks to manage change that affects the RN's practice environment
- Mobilize a variety of resources to proactively effect change in the practice environment
- Evaluate effectiveness of change within the practice environment
- Analyze data sources to establish priorities for change relevant to system needs/aims

Facilitator of Learning: Taking Professional Accountability Beyond the Bedside

- Apply principles of learning assessment in the clinical setting
- Adapt traditional teaching methods to achieve patient/family learning in atypical situations
- Identify valid and reliable approaches for evaluating outcomes of instruction

The Ripple Effect: Caring for People of Many Cultures

- Assess one's individual level of cultural IQ
- Define cultural competence
- Identify a minimum of two reasons why cultural competence is vital to the organization's future
- Identify three ways that cultural competence can impact treatment or care processes

Code of Ethics for Nurses with Interpretive Statements (American Nurses Association)

- Identify the nine planks of the Code of Ethics for Nurses
- Analyze the key interpretive statements
- Explain the significance of the Code of Ethics for Nurses in guiding and empowering nurses in their practice (empowered caring)
- Apply the Code of Ethics for Nurses to one's nursing practice and to the practice of nursing within the workplace

Summary

Given the current demands of the health-care environment, the need for nurses minimally competent with respect to behaviors/characteristics around clinical judgment, clinical inquiry, caring practices, response to diversity, advocacy/moral agency, facilitation of learning, collaboration, and systems thinking is critical in light of ever-increasing contextual complexity and variability of patient needs. The Synergy Model provides an exemplary and relevant framework for clinical practice with the ultimate aim of improving patient outcomes. Tenets of accountability and professionalism are central to the model and, in its entirety, it provides a practical and useful approach for thinking about and redesigning educational products and processes in clinical settings.

The Study of Practice: Validating Synergy

14

Sandra Greenberg, PhD, Patricia M. Muenzen, MA, and I. Leon Smith, PhD

The AACN Synergy Model for Patient Care™ is a patient-driven conceptual framework for nursing. The basic premise of the model is that optimal outcomes can be produced through the synergistic interaction between the needs of the patient and the competencies of the nurse (Curley, 1996, 1998). Such a model represents a reconceptualized view of nursing practice and would, if validated, require a uniquely designed credentialing program for practitioners. Also, implementation of the model would require revised collaborative initiatives in regard to preservice, inservice, and continuing education.

Synergy occurs, and optimal outcomes may result, when the competencies of the nurse complement the needs of the patient. Implicit in the interactions between patients and nurses is the notion that the patients with the greatest level of need require the nurses with the highest degree of competency. When nurses perform at the level of competency required to meet the needs of the patient, optimal outcomes are more likely to occur.

In 1996, AACN Certification Corporation contracted with Professional Examination Service (PES) to undertake a comprehensive, systematic study of critical care nursing practice using the Synergy Model as the conceptual framework. While the immediate objective of the study was to further articulate the components of the Synergy Model, the longer-term objectives were to facilitate the development of a model-based credentialing program for nurses providing care to acute and critically ill patients—a comprehensive credentialing program that is responsive to changes in the delivery of service to acute and critical care patients by direct care nurses and advanced practitioners.

Traditional Versus Model-Based Role Delineation

Traditional role delineation studies focus on identifying domains of practice and discrete tasks performed in a profession and the knowledge and skill base required to perform those tasks. The knowledge and skills identified in such studies becomes the focus of certification examination questions. In 1991, PES completed a traditional role delineation study of critical care nursing practice (Niebuhr, 1993). In that study, subject-matter experts (SMEs) delineated and validated the domains of practice and specific tasks performed in critical care nursing practice, together with the associated knowledge and skills. Eight body systems (e.g., cardiovascular, respiratory) provided the context for the delineation of more than 75 patient care problems. The final blueprint provided specific guidance regarding both content and process; test specifications were published in terms of percentages of questions related to the systems, patient care problems, and the associated knowledge and skills.

Consistent with the vision statement of the AACN Certification Corporation, a unique study of practice was designed to identify and validate the range of competencies required to meet the needs of acute and critically ill patients. In contrast to the traditional role delineation approach that identifies discrete knowledge and skills suitable for testing in a certification examination, a study of practice based on the Synergy Model would create a different framework for examination development and would represent a shift in focus from specific knowledge and skills to more integrated competencies.

Purpose of Study

The purpose of the study was to explore the utility of the Synergy Model in light of its potential as a guiding force in the credentialing programs implemented by the AACN Certification Corporation. Accordingly, the Synergy Model and the study of practice were viewed as ways to understand critically ill patients and critical care nurses in order to define and implement more useful eligibility, examination, and experience requirements for the changing world of the critical care nurse.

Three research questions were developed:

1. Can a set of patient characteristics be developed that comprehensively describes the patients seen by nurses providing direct care services to subacute, acute, and critically ill patients? Can patients presenting with varying levels of acuity (as globally identified by nurses) be differentiated in regard to their level of need in terms of the patient characteristics?

2. Can a set of nurse characteristics be developed that comprehensively describes the competencies of nurses providing direct care services to subacute, acute, and critically ill patients? Do nurses working with patients on the extreme ends of the patient characteristic continua identify themselves as more competent or less competent than other nurses?

3. Is there a relationship between the characteristics of the patients and the required characteristics of the nurses? That is, do nurses identify that more competent nurses are required to provide optimal outcomes to more compromised patients?

Method

Operationally Defining the Elements in the Synergy Model

Working from the preliminary think-tank conceptualization, a panel of subject-matter experts (SMEs) characterized the patient need aspect of the model in terms of eight patient characteristics—stability, complexity, predictability, resiliency, vulnerability, participation in decision-making, participation in care, and resource availability. They characterized the nurse competency aspect of the model in terms of eight nurse characteristics—clinical judgment, clinical inquiry, caring practices, response to diversity, agency/moral advocacy, facilitation of learning, collaboration, and systems thinking.

Over the course of three meetings, the SME group developed and refined definitions for the eight patient characteristics and eight nurse characteristics, and 5-point rating scales were devised to behaviorally anchor the endpoints and midpoint of the continuum describing each patient and nurse characteristic. The work of the SMEs was augmented by information obtained via critical incidents interviews and independent reviews of the definitions and the rating scales by critical care nurses and advanced-practice nurses working with acute and critically ill patients.

The 5-point rating scales for the patient characteristics were developed to include descriptors for the most compromised patients (scale point 1) and least compromised patients (scale point 5), as well as for midpoint patients (scale point 3). (See Table 14.1 for a sample of the descriptors at each of three scale points for the patient characteristic of Resiliency.) Similarly, each nurse characteristic rating scale included descriptors reflecting novice (scale point 1), competent (scale point 3), and expert (scale point 5) performance by a nurse providing direct care to a patient—consistent with the pattern of skill acquisition described by Benner (1984). (See Table 14.2 for a sample of the descriptors associated with the nurse characteristic of clinical judgment.) The sets of scales were designed so that the most critical patients would be categorized by low ratings (i.e., scale points 1 and 2) on the patient characteristics scales and the least critical patients would be categorized by high ratings (i.e., scale points 4 and 5). The directionality of the nurse characteristic scales was such that less-expert nurses would be categorized by low ratings (i.e., scale points 1 and 2) and more-expert nurses would be categorized by high ratings (i.e., scale points 4 and 5) on the nurse characteristics scales.

Table 14.1. Levels of the Patient Characteristic of Resiliency.

Level	Description
1	*Minimally resilient* Unable to mount a response Failure of compensatory/coping mechanisms Minimal reserves Brittle
3	*Moderately resilient* Able to mount a moderate response Able to initiate some degree of compensation Moderate reserves
5	*Highly resilient* Able to mount and maintain a response Intact compensatory/coping mechanisms Strong reserves Endurance

Table 14.2. Levels of the Nurse Characteristic of Clinical Judgment.

Level	Description
1	• Collects basic-level data. • Follows algorithms, decision trees, and protocols with all populations and is uncomfortable deviating from them. • Matches formal knowledge with clinical events to make decisions. • Questions the limits of one's ability to make clinical decisions and delegates the decision-making to other clinicians. • Includes extraneous detail.
3	• Collects and interprets complex patient data. • Makes clinical judgments based on an immediate grasp of the whole picture for common or routine patient populations. • Recognizes patterns and trends that may predict the direction of illness. • Recognizes limits and seeks appropriate help. • Focuses on key elements of case, while sorting out extraneous details.
5	• Synthesizes and interprets multiple, sometimes conflicting, sources of data. • Makes judgments based on an immediate grasp of the whole picture, unless working with new patient populations; uses past experiences to anticipate problems. • Helps patient and family see the "big picture." • Recognizes the limits of clinical judgment and seeks multidisciplinary collaboration and consultation with comfort. • Recognizes and responds to the dynamic situation.

Instrumentation and Procedures

A survey instrument was developed to gather data to address the three research questions. The survey contained three major sections, each directed toward an examination of one question, plus a background questionnaire and section soliciting qualitative comments about the Synergy Model.

In the first section of the survey, respondents were asked to review each patient characteristic and its associated 5-point rating scale, then indicate the percentage of their own patients who functioned at each point on the scale. The specific question posed was:

> Consider all of the patients in your primary employment setting to whom you provided direct care in the last thirty (30) days. **Think of the time when their needs were the greatest.** Then, regardless of the actual number of patients you saw, write down the percentage of those patients who could be described by Levels 1, 2, 3, 4, and 5.

Given the directionality of the scales, it was expected that nurses caring for more-compromised patients would indicate that a higher percentage of their patients function at the lower scale points; conversely, nurses caring for less-compromised patients would indicate that a higher percentage of their patients function at the higher scale points.

In the second section of the survey, respondents were asked to review each nurse characteristic, then indicate where their own performance fell on the associated 5-point scale. Specifically, they were asked to select the level that represented a self-assessment of their own level of performance on each nurse characteristic. It was thought that nurses working with more-compromised patients might identify themselves as performing at higher levels of competency than would nurses working with less-compromised patients.

The third section of the survey was designed to provide an indirect exploration of the basic premise of the Synergy Model: that optimal outcomes are achieved when nursing competencies are matched to patient needs. It was reasoned that, given the goal of achieving optimal patient outcomes, more-compromised patients would be identified as requiring direct care nurses performing at higher levels of competency on each nurse characteristic than would less-compromised patients. Therefore, when nurses were presented with descriptions of patients ranging from subacute to critically ill, it was hypothesized that they would identify differentiated levels of nursing competency as required to achieve optimal outcomes.

To address the question, SMEs developed patient profiles, structured as nurse-to-nurse shift change reports. Each profile included a review of systems, laboratory values, medication orders, psychosocial information, and an overview of the patient's status. Assignments for profile development were made such that each SME was responsible for the development of one profile of a neonatal, pediatric, or adult patient at a particular level of criticality (low, medium, or high). During the development process, other SMEs reviewed the profiles and provided feedback on the degree to which the profile fit the assignment. Box 14.1 contains a patient profile for an adult, acutely ill patient, and Box 14.2 contains a patient profile for a pediatric, critically ill patient.

Box 14.1. Adult Acute Care Patient Profile

Rose is a 65-year-old woman with shortness of breath that has been increasing for the past few weeks. She has a long-time history of exertional dyspnea, but recently she is breathless even at rest. She had an aortic valve replacement 18 years ago. Also, she has a history of rheumatic fever, hypertension, CHF, and diabetes controlled with diet.

Four days ago she came into the emergency department. She had wheezing, crackles (rales) one third of the way up, and hepatomegaly.

Chest x-ray showed pulmonary edema. She received furosemide (Lasix) and responded with a good urine output. Rose was admitted to the CICU for pulmonary edema. While in the CICU, she had an echocardiogram that revealed mild left ventricular hypertrophy, severe aortic stenosis, and a 55% ejection fraction. It was decided to redo the aortic valve replacement.

She had her surgery yesterday and has had an unstable night. The major problems have been a low urine output and low mean arterial pressure (MAP). She is on dobutamine (Dobutrex), 6mcg/kg/min, and neo-synephrine has just been added to increase her MAP to 70–75.

Review of Systems

Cardiopulmonary

She has been in sinus tachycardia with MAP ranging from 59 to 64. There are two mediastinal tubes and two pleural tubes with a minimal amount of drainage. Overnight, her hemodynamic values were: CVP = 5–8; PAP = 36/12–38/15; CI = 4.2–5.2; PVR = 587; SVR = 600. Rose's skin is pale and warm, extremities are warm, and she appears puffy.

Respiratory

She is intubated with an oral 7.5 ET tube. The ventilator is set at 100% F_IO_2; V_T 550; IMV = 10; PEEP = 5. Her SaO_2 is ranging from 97 to 99%. During the night she desaturated to 82% so the F_IO_2 was increased to its present 100%. Her current ABGs are PaO_2 = 399; CO_2 = 46; pH = 7.32; HCO_3 = 23; O_2 Saturation = 99%. We are going to decrease her to 80% F_IO_2. Her respiratory rate has been 10 most of the night. Breath sounds are equal with bilateral scattered rhonchi that clear after suctioning. She was suctioned three times, the last time at 0630 for a moderate amount of thin clear secretions.

Gastrointestinal

Her nasogastric tube has drained 200 ml of dark-green drainage. Her abdomen is soft, but no bowel sounds were heard.

Neurological

Pupils are midposition with a brisk response to both direct and consensual light. Cough and gag reflex are present. She moves all extremities to commands and opens her eyes when her name is called. She has slept most of the night.

Renal

BUN = 20; creatinine = 2.4

Her output has been 120 ml for the past 8 hours. I gave her Lasix, 240 mg around 0200 with minimal response. Her attending physician started the Neo-synephrine to increase her MAP to 70–75, because she may need higher filling pressure to perfuse her kidneys.

Hematology

RBCs = 3.02 million/mm^3

WBCs = 29,200/mm^3

Hemoglobin = 9.7 g/dl

Her temperature has been low-grade at 100.4 F (38 C). They just ordered her to have blood, urine, and sputum cultures because of her high WBC count.

IV Fluids/Drips/Electrolytes:

Maintenance fluids = D5/1/4 NS at 10cc

Nitroglycerin, 25 mcg/min

Neo-synephrine, 50 mcg/min

Dobutamine 6 mcg/kg/min

0600 laboratory results are: Na = 134; K = 4.9; Cl = 104; BS = 200 with 5 unit regular insulin at 0700

Skin

She has no skin breakdown. Her mediastinal dressing is dry and intact.

Vascular Access

She has a right internal jugular pulmonary artery catheter; two PIVs one in the right hand and one in the left forehand. She has a right radial arterial line.

Social

Rose has been married for 40 years. Her husband is a retired auto worker with excellent health-care benefits. They have lived together in their present ranch style house for the past 30 years. They have two children who are married and have two children each. They were all here yesterday after the surgery, and her husband called today around 0600.

Team

Dr. X is Rose's cardiologist; Dr. Y is the cardiac surgeon who performed the surgery.

Summary

Rose is a 65-year-old woman status post redo of an aortic valve replacement. Her vital signs have remained constant through the night. Her MAP remains at 63 mm Hg, and I have continued to increase the neo-synephrine. Her urine output has remained at 10–20 ml per hour. The team feels that if the MAP can be maintained at 70–75 mm Hg, her urine output will improve. She will remain ventilated today with concentration on weaning the FiO_2.

Box 14.2. Pediatric Critical Care Patient Profile

Ann is a 5-year-old girl who suffered a full cardiopulmonary arrest yesterday in the emergency department (ED) after presenting in shock after a 2-day history of fever, vomiting, and abdominal pain. She has a positive medical history—hospitalized 2.5 years ago with idiopathic dilated cardiomyopathy that responded well to therapy. She was off all medications (digoxin, diuretics, and enalapril) and was considered to be in excellent health 2 weeks before in cardiology clinic.

Pre-arrest in the ED, she was poorly perfused and lethargic but able to respond appropriately. Quick look echocardiogram (ECHO) revealed severe systolic left-ventricular (LV) dysfunction. Post-arrest, she was unable to sustain an adequate blood pressure with maximal conventional therapy, so she was emergently transferred to the intensive care unit (ICU) and placed on extracorporeal membrane oxygenation (ECMO).

The working diagnosis is profound cardiac failure of questionable etiology. The plan is to maintain ECMO support and consider cardiac transplantation if her neurological evaluation is reasonable.

She had an unstable night; the major problem has been bleeding from her ECMO cannula sites.

She was re-explored twice but continues with 80-100 mL of chest tube drainage per hour.

Blood bank has been able to keep up with her losses, providing continuous replacement of packed cells, 5% albumin, FFP, platelets, and cryoprecipitate.
She is on Amicar continuous infusion at 750 mg/hr (per ECMO protocol).

Review of Systems and Current Orders

Cardiopulmonary

She is on ECMO with an open chest and 3 transthoracic cannulas: 2 venous (1 RA & 1 LA) and 1 arterial return to the aorta.

She has an occlusive transparent dressing over her open chest.

Ann's skin is still pale and mottled; capillary refill is 4-5 sec; extremities are cool and she appears puffy; has periorbital edema.

Overnight, our goal has been to keep her MAPs around 70 mmHg, RAP <15 mmHg and LAP <10 mmHg by increasing ECMO flow as much as possible; with volume replacement; and by manipulating epinephrine, dopamine, and amrinone.

Because of inadequate venous cannula size, we've been unable to increase her flow more than 1.8 L/min. The cardiac surgeons would like to replace her RA cannula with a larger size later this morning.

We've kept up with her mediastinal drainage—replacing cc per cc. You have to stay on top of her 3 mediastinal drains because they clot easily.

Ann was initially hypotensive, with MAPs in the 50s, but she weaned off epinephrine by midnight then weaned to renal dose (2.5 mcg/kg/min) dopamine by 2 a.m. At 4 a.m. cardiology recommended that we start amrinone for afterload reduction; she's now on 5 mcg/kg/min—they also discussed nitroglycerin, which may be used later.

Ann has been in normal sinus rhythm/sinus tachycardia (NSR/ST) most of the night.

She did have a short period of ventricular fibrillation (VF) during her first exploration but easily converted to NSR with 20 joules using internal paddles.

After that we bolused her with Lidocaine 20mg, then started a Lidocaine drip at 20 mcg/kg/min.

She has had no spontaneous arrhythmias since; 06:00 Lidocaine level = 2.04. Given her contractility, they might want to discontinue this.

She has A&V wires in place; the pacemaker captures easily but we haven't needed it.

She is intubated with an oral 5.0 mm cuffed ET tube—cuff is down.

She is on 25/5, 0.6 F_IO_2 at a rate of 10; the high F_IO_2 is for coronary artery perfusion.

Breath sounds are equal with bilateral scattered rhonchi that clear somewhat after suctioning.

She was suctioned twice—last time was at 5 a.m. for a scant amount of thin white secretions.

Last set of gases: arterial 7.47/34/314/24/100% and mixed venous 7.42/40/42/25/79%.

Parameters have changed all night—check to see what is decided on rounds.

Hematology

Hct: 23.7; PT 16.2; Platelets 129K; Fibrinogen 187.

Heparin requirements have decreased overnight—ACTs currently 200.

Her evolving coagulopathy may be due to sepsis.

Infectious Disease

We're keeping her temperature at 95° fahrenheit (35° celsius) to decrease metabolic requirements.

Full cultures were sent yesterday—nothing preliminary thus far.

She is on triple antibiotic coverage.

Fluids, Electrolytes, and Nutrition

Maintenance fluids D5/0.25% NS with 10mEq KCl at 30 mL/hr

Potassium bolus x 2 for K$^+$ level of 3.0; Calcium gluconate bolus x 1 for Cal 8.9

06:00 labs: Na 147; K 3.2; Cl 94; TCO$_2$ 32; BS 152; Ical 0.94; Cal 8.6; Phos 5.5; Mg 2.2; TP 5.8; Alb 2.8

Need to order TPN/Lipids today.

Neurological

Pupils are midposition with a sluggish response to both direct and consensual light—last dose of atropine received about 18 hours ago.

No cough, gag, corneals, or doll's eyes.

No spontaneous movement.

+ 4 thumb abduction to train-of-four stimulation—no pavulon since cannulation yesterday.

Her lowest pH during her arrest was 6.99.

Neurology will see her today (baseline: doing well in kindergarten).

Comfort: Receiving 1.5 mg/hr of morphine; may consider lorazepam q8hrs and midazolam prn.

Renal

BUN 48; creatinine 1.7

No urine output—foley irrigated with normal saline—bladder not palpable.

Bolus x 1 with furosemide without diuresis.

ICU attending mentioned a continuous furosemide infusion—check with renal.

Renal team will consult today—anticipate CVVH/dialysis via the ECMO circuit tomorrow.

Gastrointestinal

No bowel sounds; nasogastric tube (NGT) to suction; 100mL bilious Heme + drainage.

On ranitidine.

Skin

She has a jell pad under her occiput.

On an Effica CC bed at 5ft—no turns with open chest.

Ask the specialty bed company to send in their CNS for a bed adjustment.

Vascular access

She has more than adequate access.

Pressors and sedation are going into the circuit.

You can use the RA for blood products; LA is transduced.

She has a right double-lumen femoral.

She has a right radial A-line that draws well.

Social

Ann is 5 years old and is the third of four children. The other children are ages 11, 7, and 3 months. Parents are married and live together. Dad is a fireman and mom is a teacher but currently on maternity leave.

Parents are upset. Both are here and aware of her status. Both have seen her recently. They, especially Dad, can only stay at the bedside for a few minutes before they have to leave. Mom is able to ask questions and appears to be processing information. The other children are in their aunt's care—there is a large extended family.

Team

Dr. X is Ann's cardiologist; Dr. X is on for heart transplant; X is the on call nurse.

Dr. X is the cardiac surgeon; Dr. X is the fellow; Dr. X is the ICU physician; Dr. X is on for ECMO; Dr. X is on for neurology; and Dr. X is on for the renal team. Primary care physician is Dr. X, who appears to have a very good relationship with the parents.

Summary Statement

Ann is a 5-year-old female, status post cardiopulmonary arrest of unclear etiology. The team is hopeful that she has reversible single organ (cardiac) failure. If not reversible and only single system (no neurological sequelae), she will be listed for heart transplant. Ann is extremely sensitive to even slight physiological changes and requires moment-to-moment vigilant monitoring and reciprocal interventions to manage her tenuous status. Her medical team is very large, and it has been very difficult to develop and maintain one cohesive unifying plan. Ann's family is devastated, but everyone appears mutually supportive. The team has been communicating well with the family.

In the third section of the survey, respondents were asked to rate three hypothetical patients representing different points on the criticality continuum—low, medium, and high. No information was provided regarding the theoretical criticality level of the patients—that is, whether the patients were supposed to be functioning at a low, medium, or high criticality level. Respondents rated each patient using the patient characteristic rating scales, assigning a level 1, 2, 3, 4, or 5 for each patient characteristic, and made an overall rating of the patient's level of criticality using a 5-point scale. Then, for each of the three patients, they were asked to indicate the level of competency that a nurse would need to demonstrate on each nurse characteristic (i.e., level 1, 2, 3, 4, or 5) in order to achieve optimal outcomes for that patient.

Data Collection

Table 14.3 provides a summary of the elements of the survey and the data collected. The survey instrument was sent to a sample of 3,975 registered nurses: 2,000 nurses of adult patients, 1,150 nurses of pediatric patients, and 825 nurses of neonatal patients. One-half of the nurses providing care to patients in each age category were critical care nurses drawn from the AACN Certification Corporation's membership database, and one-half were acute care and/or subacute care nurses whose names were drawn from relevant journal subscription mailing lists. The members of the sample received a survey containing three patient profiles consistent with the age of their own patients.

Table 14.3. Survey Ratings.

Section	Task
1	Respondents were asked to consider all of the patients in their primary employment setting to whom they provided care in the last 30 days, to think of the time when their needs were the greatest, and to write down the percentage of those patients who could be described by Levels 1, 2, 3, 4, and 5 on each patient characteristic. Level 1 represented the least positive aspect of a patient characteristic and Level 5 represented the most positive aspect of a patient characteristic.
2	Respondents were asked to circle the level (1, 2, 3, 4 or 5) that represents a self-assessment of their own level of performance on each nurse characteristic. Level 1 described an entry-level nurse and Level 5 described an expert nurse.
3	Respondents read three profiles, or write-ups of actual nurse-to-nurse shift change reports. The profiles included examples of low, medium, and high criticality patients. Respondents rated each patient using the patient characteristic rating scales. When they had completed their ratings for each patient characteristic, they were asked to make an overall judgment of how critically ill they believed that patient to be, using a 1-to-5 scale. Then, for each nurse characteristic, they were asked to rate the level of performance that a nurse would need to display to meet the patient's needs and facilitate optimal outcomes for him.

Section	Task
4	This section elicited professional and background information such as respondent's patient population, work setting, education, years of experience, etc.
5	This section solicited open-ended comments regarding characteristics of patients or nurses that might be missing from the Synergy Model.

Participants received a sequence of three mailings: a letter inviting them to participate in the upcoming survey; the survey mailing including the survey instrument, a resource book containing the patient and nurse rating scales, and an application to receive 1.5 hours of continuing education credit for their participation; and a follow-up postcard thanking them for completing the survey.

Eight hundred seventy-one completed surveys were returned out of 3,557 eligible, for an overall response rate of 24%. Respondents had an average of 14 years of experience in nursing. The majority (75%) of respondents were staff nurses, 11% were charge nurses, and less than 5% each were managers, clinical nurse specialists, nurse practitioners, case managers, nurse consultants, or nurse educators.

Data Analysis

In preparation for data analysis, each respondent was classified as either a neonatal, pediatric, or adult nurse on the basis of the response to a background question regarding the percentage of a respondent's patients falling within each age range. Each respondent also was classified as a subacute care, acute care, or critical care nurse on the basis of the responses to a background question regarding the percentage of their patients falling within each acuity level. Assignment was made by creating a composite score, or weighted average, of the percentage of their patients the respondent judged to be functioning at each of these three acuity levels. Patient acuity classification scores ranged from 1 to 5. Nurses with higher percentages of critically ill patients had lower patient classification scores, and nurses with lower percentages of critically ill patients had higher patient classification scores. In absolute terms, the patient acuity classification scores used to assign each nurses to a patient population classification were as follows: 1 – 2.0 = critical care nurse, 2.1 – 3.9 = acute care nurse, and 4.0 – 5 = subacute care nurse.

Finally, for each respondent, the percentage distribution of the respondent's patients across all five scale points of a given patient characteristic was transformed into a composite score for that patient characteristic. Patient characteristic composite scores ranged from 1 to 5. Lower patient characteristic composite scores indicated that a higher percentage of that nurse's patients functioned at the more compromised end of the patient characteristic rating scale, and higher composite scores indicated that a lower percentage of that nurse's patients functioned at the more compromised end of the rating scale.

Results

Patient Characteristics

Relationship to perceived patient acuity. Examination of frequency distributions for each patient characteristic showed that nurses did use all five scale points when describing their patients. Nurses working in intensive care units (ICUs) indicated that the majority of their patients functioned at the more compromised end of each patient characteristic rating scale, but did describe some of their patients as functioning at less compromised levels. Nurses working in nonintensive care units indicated that the majority of their patients functioned at the less compromised end of each patient characteristic rating scale, but did describe some of their patients as functioning at more compromised levels. Exploration of the qualitative comments regarding the eight patient characteristics suggests that the characteristics provide a thorough description of patients.

Mean patient characteristic composite scores were calculated separately for nurses working with neonatal, pediatric, and adult patient populations. Within each patient population, patient characteristic composite scores were calculated separately for nurses who had been classified as subacute care, acute care, or critical care. The results are displayed in Table 14.4. Composite scores exhibited the expected pattern. That is, for each of 24 possible comparisons, nurses classified as caring primarily for subacute care patients characterized their patients as more stable, less complex, more predictable, more resilient, less vulnerable, more able to participate in decision-making and care, and having greater resource availability than nurses classified as caring primarily for acutely ill patients. Moreover, for 23 of 24 possible comparisons, nurses who were classified as caring primarily for acute care patients on the basis of their demographic questionnaire characterized their patients as functioning at the higher end of the patient characteristic rating scales than did nurses classified as caring primarily for critically-ill patients. The data suggest that the eight patient characteristics differentiate the patients of nurses who describe their patient populations as differing in acuity.

Table 14.4. Mean Patient Characteristic Ratings by Nurses Classified by Age and Acuity of Patient Population.

Patient Characteristic	Neonatal			Pediatric			Adult		
	Subacute	Acute	Critical	Subacute	Acute	Critical	Subacute	Acute	Critical
Stability									
M*	3.8	3.1	2.7	4.2	3.6	2.7	3.4	3.1	2.8
SD*		1.0	1.0	0.9	0.7	0.9	0.6	1.0	0.7
N*	33	43	131	40	45	78	88	136	155
Complexity									
M	3.5	2.8	2.2	3.3	2.8	2.4	3.1	2.8	2.4
SD	1.0	1.0	0.9	1.1	1.0	0.6	1.0	0.8	0.7
N	33	43	132	39	45	78	88	137	155
Predictability									
M	4.2	3.5	3.3	4.0	3.6	3.3	3.7	3.6	3.3
SD	0.7	0.9	1.0	0.8	0.8	0.7	0.8	0.7	0.8
N	33	43	132	40	45	78	88	137	155
Resiliency									
M	3.5	2.9	2.5	3.6	3.3	2.8	3.2	2.9	2.6
SD	1.1	1.1	0.9	1.0	0.9	0.7	0.9	0.7	0.6
N	33	43	130	40	45	78	88	137	155
Vulnerability									
M	2.9	2.4	2.0	3.1	2.8	2.5	3.0	2.6	2.4
SD	1.1	1.0	0.8	1.1	0.9	0.7	0.9	0.7	0.6
N	33	43	131	40	45	78	88	146	156
Participation in Decision-Making									
M	3.7	3.6	3.4	3.8	3.7	3.5	3.6	3.5	3.4
SD	0.9	0.9	1.0	1.0	0.7	0.6	0.8	0.7	0.8
N	33	43	131	40	45	77	87	147	155
Participation in Care									
M	3.9	3.6	3.3	3.7	3.6	3.2	3.4	3.2	2.9
SD	0.7	0.8	0.9	1.0	0.8	0.7	0.9	0.8	0.8
N	32	43	132	40	45	78	87	137	155

Patient Characteristic	Neonatal			Pediatric			Adult		
	Subacute	Acute	Critical	Subacute	Acute	Critical	Subacute	Acute	Critical
Resource Availability									
M	3.2	2.9	2.9	3.3	3.2	3.0	3.2	3.1	3.0
SD	1.1	0.8	1.0	1.1	0.8	0.9	0.9	0.7	0.8
N	32	43	131	40	45	78	88	137	155

M = Mean; SD = Standard Deviation; N = Number.

A multivariate trend analysis confirmed the relationship between patient acuity and patient characteristic composite scores reported in Table 14.5. For each patient population (neonatal, pediatric, and adult), there was a strong and significant linear association between patient acuity scores (derived from nurses' estimates of the percentage of their patients who could be described as subacute care, acute care and critical care) and composite scores for six of the eight patient characteristics (i.e., stability, complexity, predictability, resiliency, vulnerability, and participation in care). Nurses who described their patient population as more acute also rated the patients they had seen in the past month as less stable, less resilient, less predictable, more vulnerable, and less able to participate in care than nurses who rated their patient populations as less acute. Nurses who described their patient population as less acute based on the demographic questionnaire also rated their patients as more stable, more predictable, more resilient, less vulnerable, and more able to participate in care.

Table 14.5. MANOVA: Trend Analysis of Patient Characteristic Ratings Made by Nurses Working With Neonatal, Pediatric, and Adult Patient Populations.

Effect	df	F	t-value							
			RE	VU	ST	CO	RA	PC	PD	PR
Neonatal		3.5								
Linear	1		5.0*	5.1*	5.6*	6.9*	1.8	3.2*	1.3	4.8*
Quadratic	1		0.4	0.2	0.5	0.0	1.2	0.4	0.1	1.1
Pediatric		5.4								

Effect	df	F	t-value							
			RE	VU	ST	CO	RA	PC	PD	PR
Linear	1		4.6*	3.6*	9.8*	5.3*	1.6	3.0*	1.9	5.0*
Quadratic	1		-0.8	-0.3	-1.5	-0.1	-0.4	-1.2	-0.7	0.4
Adult		4.7								
Linear	1		5.4*	6.1*	5.8*	6.4*	1.5	4.1*	0.8	3.4*
Quadratic	1		0.5	1.0	-0.5	0.0	0.5	-0.1	-0.4	0.2

RE = Resiliency; VU = Vulnerability; ST = Stability; CO = Complexity; RA = Resource Availability; PC = Participation in Care; PD = Participation in Decision-Making; PR = Predictability.

Relationships among the patient characteristics. Intercorrelations among the patient characteristic composite scores were also explored (see Table 14.6). For each patient population, correlations among the patient characteristics ranged from .15 to .68, suggesting modest relationships among the patient characteristics. An exploratory factor analysis (maximum likelihood with varimax rotation) was conducted to further explore these relationships (see Table 14.7). A two-factor solution was obtained for each of the three patient age groups. For nurses of neonatal and pediatric patients, the first factor consisted of stability, complexity, predictability, resiliency, and vulnerability. This factor seems to reflect the intrinsic (e.g., internal, physiological) characteristics of the patient and family. The second factor consisted of participation in decision-making, participation in care, and resource availability. This factor seems to reflect characteristics extrinsic (e.g., external, contextual) to the patient and family. A similar two-factor solution emerged for the adult group, with the exception that predictability loaded with the extrinsic characteristics, rather than the intrinsic characteristics.

Table 14.6. Correlations Among the Patient Characteristics.

	RE	VU	ST	CO	RA	PC	PD	PR
Neonatal								
Resiliency	—							
Vulnerability	.66	—						
Stability	.68	.65	—					
Complexity	.57	.64	.64	—				
Resource Availability	.26	.25	.30	.26	—			
Participation in Care	.44	.35	.42	.42	.54	—		

	RE	VU	ST	CO	RA	PC	PD	PR
Participation in Decision-Making	.32	.27	.36	.29	.45	.64	—	
Predictability	.51	.43	.56	.44	.25	.41	.37	—

Pediatric

	RE	VU	ST	CO	RA	PC	PD	PR
Resiliency	—							
Vulnerability	.49	—						
Stability	.64	.54	—					
Complexity	.40	.48	.56	—				
Resource Availability	.29	.35	.27	.30	—			
Participation in Care	.46	.43	.47	.39	.47	—		
Participation in Decision-Making	.26	.38	.24	.32	.49	.60	—	
Predictability	.57	.46	.62	.47	.15	.37	.21	—

Adult

	RE	VU	ST	CO	RA	PC	PD	PR
Resiliency	—							
Vulnerability	.52	—						
Stability	.60	.56	—					
Complexity	.39	.52	.56	—				
Resource Availability	.27	.28	.30	.27	—			
Participation in Care	.38	.32	.38	.25	.50	—		
Participation in Decision-Making	.35	.28	.43	.24	.40	.52	—	
Predictability	.38	.30	.49	.38	.30	.37	.47	—

RE = Resiliency; VU = Vulnerability; ST = Stability; CO = Complexity; RA = Resource Availability; PC = Participation in Care; PD = Participation in Decision Making; PR = Predictability.

Table 14.7. Factor Analysis of Patient Characteristics.

Patient Characteristic	Neonatal		Pediatric		Adult	
	Factor 1	Factor 2	Factor 1	Factor 2	Factor 1	Factor 2
Resiliency	.76	.26	.71	.23	.63	.31
Vulnerability	.79	.15	.57	.37	.67	.21
Stability	.80	.26	.83	.18	.78	.32

Patient Characteristic	Neonatal		Pediatric		Adult	
	Factor 1	Factor 2	Factor 1	Factor 2	Factor 1	Factor 2
Complexity	.72	.24	.57	.30	.66	.16
Resource Availability	.17	.58	.19	.59	.18	.57
Participation in Care	.29	.81	.40	.66	.21	.72
Participation in Decision Making	.20	.70	.12	.82	.25	.67
Predictability	.54	.32	.73	.13	.42	.44

The findings from the trend analysis also support the distinction between the intrinsic and extrinsic nurse characteristics. While all five of the intrinsic characteristics bore a linear relationship with patient acuity scores, only one of the three extrinsic characteristics (participation in care) did so. Thus, it appears that the intrinsic characteristics are more closely tied to nurses' perceptions of the overall acuity of their patients.

Exploration of the qualitative comments regarding the completeness of the set of patient characteristics suggests that respondents perceive that the eight characteristics provide a thorough description of important patient variables.

Self-Ratings on the Nurse Characteristics

Descriptive statistics for nurse characteristic self-ratings are presented in Table 14.8. Self-ratings were high for all eight nurse characteristics; on average, respondents placed themselves toward the expert end of the continuum. Correlations between years of experience and nurse self-ratings revealed that more experienced nurses rated themselves higher on each nurse characteristic than did less experienced nurses.

Table 14.8. Means, Standard Deviations, and Correlations Among the Nurse Self-Ratings.

Nurse Characteristic	M	SD	CJ	MA	CP	CL	ST	RD	CI	FL
Clinical Judgment	4.3	0.7	—							
Advocacy/Moral Agency	3.9	0.8	.37	—						
Caring Practices	4.2	0.8	.39	.42	—					
Collaboration	4.2	0.8	.48	.37	.36	—				
Systems Thinking	4.0	0.8	.45	.47	.44	.38	—			
Nurse Characteristic	M	SD	CJ	MA	CP	CL	ST	RD	CI	FL
Response to Diversity	4.0	0.8	.24	.29	.31	.25	.38	—		
Clinical Inquiry	4.0	0.9	.51	.41	.33	.49	.40	.38	—	
Facilitator of Learning	4.0	0.9	.30	.32	.42	.33	.46	.46	.43	—

M = Mean; SD = Standard Deviations; CJ = Clinical Judgment; MA = Advocacy/Moral Agency; CP = Caring Practices; CL = Collaboration; ST = Systems Thinking; RD = Response to Diversity; CI = Clinical Inquiry; FL = Facilitator of Learning.

T-tests were conducted to compare the mean self-ratings of subgroups of nurses. Nurses based in intensive care units (where patients tend to be more compromised) rated themselves higher on the nurse characteristics of clinical judgment, clinical inquiry, collaboration, and systems thinking than did nurses in non-intensive care settings (where patients tend to be less compromised). Regardless of unit or setting, self-ratings on the nurse characteristics of clinical judgment, clinical inquiry, collaboration, and systems thinking were modestly correlated with the patient acuity scores. These findings suggest that nurses who characterize their patient populations as more acutely ill perceive themselves as performing at higher levels of nursing competency than do nurses who characterize their patient populations as less acutely ill.

Exploration of the qualitative comments regarding the completeness of the set of nurse characteristics suggests that respondents perceive that the eight characteristics provide a thorough description of important nurse competencies.

Results Related to the Patient Profiles

Criticality ratings. Ratings of the overall criticality of the low, medium, and high criticality patient profiles generally corresponded to the levels of criticality initially assigned by the profile developers. Accordingly, respondents tended to rate the high criticality profile as equal to or higher in overall criticality than the medium criticality profile, and to rate the medium criticality profile as equal to or higher in overall criticality than the low criticality profile.

Correspondence between rated and intended patient criticality was greatest for the pediatric patient profile set, where 98% of respondents ranked the criticality of the three patient profiles in accordance with intentions. Correspondence was lowest (72%) for the neonatal patient profile set. Where criticality ratings departed from the expected ordering, respondents tended to perceive the medium criticality neonate (a full-term boy, observed for respiratory compromise and maternal drug effects) as more critically ill than the high criticality neonate (a 28-week, premature boy with respiratory distress syndrome). The correspondence rate was 81% for the adult patient profiles. Where criticality ratings departed from the expected ordering, nurses ranked the low criticality adult (an AIDS patient who was not at a critical stage of the disease) as higher in criticality than the medium criticality adult. In the latter cases, it is possible that nurses' perceptions of the gravity of the disease colored their views of the patient's immediate status, which was not critical.

Relationship of patient characteristics to overall patient criticality. Treating each respondent's ratings for the three patients as independent observations, correlations were calculated between the patient characteristic ratings and the overall criticality ratings. Table 14.9 displays the results. The intrinsic patient characteristics were moderately to highly correlated with the overall evaluation of patient criticality, while the extrinsic patient characteristics were less highly correlated with perceived overall patient criticality.

Table 14.9. Correlation Between Each Patient Characteristic and Overall Criticality.

Patient Characteristic	Neonatal	Pediatric	Adult
Resiliency	.72*	.75*	.61*
Vulnerability	.70*	.81*	.53*
Stability	.78*	.82*	.72*
Complexity	.53*	.71*	.53*
Resource Availability	.06	.33*	.28*
Participation in Care	.56*	.57*	.44*
Participation in Decision-Making	.46*	.46*	.40*
Predictability	.71*	.77*	.38*

Note. N=370 for neonatal, 552 for pediatric, 885 for adult* p<.05

Relationship between patient characteristics and nurse characteristics. Again treating each respondent's ratings for the three patients as independent observations, correlations were calculated between the nine patient ratings (patient characteristics and overall criticality ratings) and ratings of the competency of the direct care nurse providing care to the patient. Results for the neonatal, pediatric, and adult profile sets are displayed in Table 14.10.

Table 14.10. Correlations Between Patient Profile and Patient and Nurse Characteristic Ratings.

Nurse Characteristics	Patient Characteristics								
Neonatal Patient Profiles	**RE**	**VU**	**ST**	**CO**	**RA**	**PC**	**PD**	**PR**	**OC**
Clinical Judgment	-.48	-.48	-.47	-.35	.03	-.33	-.29	-.43	-.53
Agency/Moral Advocacy	-.18	-.17	-.20	-.16	-.17	.17	-.14	-.16	-.19
Caring Practices	-.32	-.35	-.30	-.26	-.03	-.20	-.20	-.28	-.35
Collaboration	-.32	-.26	-.30	-.22	-.03	-.22	-.19	-.31	-.34
Systems Thinking	-.30	-.31	-.28	-.30	-.02	-.21	-.17	-.28	-.36
Response to Diversity	-.10	-.16	-.13	-.17	-.10	-.12	-.08	-.17	-.12
Clinical Inquiry	-.32	-.33	-.35	-.23	.05	-.22	-.23	-.36	-.38
Facilitator of Learning	-.21	-.22	-.15	-.22	-.04	-.12	-.11	-.16	-.21
Pediatric Patient Profiles	**RE**	**VU**	**ST**	**CO**	**RA**	**PC**	**PD**	**PR**	**OC**
Clinical Judgment	-.52	-.54	-.54	-.55	-.22	-.31	-.27	-.50	-.61
Agency/Moral Advocacy	-.39	-.40	-.42	-.38	-.15	-.25	-.19	-.35	-.42
Caring Practices	-.36	-.36	-.38	-.37	-.17	-.21	-.16	-.36	-.39
Collaboration	-.37	-.40	-.40	-.43	-.20	-.25	-.23	-.37	-.43
Systems Thinking	-.38	-.42	-.41	-.41	-.20	-.22	-.20	-.35	-.45
Response to Diversity	-.31	-.29	-.32	-.29	-.20	-.16	-.13	-.26	-.39
Clinical Inquiry	-.41	-.41	-.43	-.41	-.22	-.21	-.18	-.39	-.50
Facilitator of Learning	-.20	-.21	-.22	-.24	-.09	-.05	-.03	-.21	-.26
Adult Patient Profiles	**RE**	**VU**	**ST**	**CO**	**RA**	**PC**	**PD**	**PR**	**OC**
Clinical Judgment	-.27	-.24	-.30	-.24	.00	-.19	-.14	-.18	-.40
Agency/Moral Advocacy	-.19	-.25	-.19	-.16	.06	.03	.01	-.01	-.09
Caring Practices	-.24	-.22	-.22	-.20	.07	-.03	-.05	-.08	-.20
Collaboration	-.20	-.21	-.14	-.15	.08	-.02	.00	-.06	-.15
Systems Thinking	-.22	-.21	-.19	-.17	.09	-.02	-.02	-.12	-.19
Response to Diversity	-.06	-.13	-.04	-.06	.13.	.11	.08	.06	.03

Nurse Characteristics	Patient Characteristics								
Adult Patient Profiles	**RE**	**VU**	**ST**	**CO**	**RA**	**PC**	**PD**	**PR**	**OC**
Clinical Inquiry	-.18	-.17	-.14	-.14	.10	-.04	-.05	-.10	-.19
Facilitator of Learning	.02	-.01	.02	-.02	.19	.13	.09	.05	.04

Note. RE=Resiliency; VU=Vulnerability; ST=Stability; CO=Complexity; RA=Resource Availability; PC=Participation in Care; PD=Participation in Decision-Making; PR=Predictability; OC=Overall Criticality.

As predicted by the model, patient characteristics and nurse characteristics were correlated in most instances. Given the directionality of the rating scales, the correlations indicate that more compromised patients were perceived to require nursing care at higher levels of the nursing competencies. The correlations were somewhat weaker for the adult patient profiles than for the neonatal and pediatric patient profiles. Across age groups, the intrinsic patient characteristics were most highly correlated with the nurse characteristics. Overall, the nurse characteristic of clinical judgment was most highly correlated with the patient characteristics, perhaps because it is best understood and most well-established in nursing literature.

An exploratory factor analysis was conducted to examine the relationships among the patient characteristic ratings for the patient profiles, and the results are displayed in Table 14.11. An identical two-factor solution was produced for the neonatal, pediatric, and adult patient profile sets: Factor 1 consisted of the intrinsic characteristics of stability, complexity, predictability, resiliency, and vulnerability; Factor 2 consisted of the extrinsic characteristics of participation in decision-making, participation in care, and resource availability. These results are similar to those obtained for the patient characteristic composite scores and further support the notion of two types of patient characteristics, the latter type highlighting an environmental or context dimension.

Table 14.11. Factor Analysis of Patient Profile and Patient Characteristic Ratings.

Patient Characteristic	Neonatal		Pediatric		Adult	
	Factor 1	Factor 2	Factor 1	Factor 2	Factor 1	Factor 2
Resiliency	.84	.18	.79	.35	.82	.25
Vulnerability	.81	.17	.82	.31	.79	.10
Stability	.82	.25	.87	.30	.75	.28
Complexity	.58	.24	.71	.33	.55	.32
Resource Availability	.04	.45	.21	.47	.20	.51

Patient Characteristic	Neonatal		Pediatric		Adult	
	Factor 1	Factor 2	Factor 1	Factor 2	Factor 1	Factor 2
Participation in Care	.48	.76	.38	.78	.22	.84
Participation in Decision-Making	.35	.88	.25	.73	.19	.80
Predictability	.70	.27	.77	.36	.36	.34

Summary

Three sets of research questions were developed and investigated. In each case, the results confirmed the expectation inherent in the Synergy Model.

1. The patient characteristics comprehensively describe the functioning (and needs) of patients seen by nurses who globally identify their patients as subacute, acute care, and critical care. Regardless of the acuity level, some patients function at each scale point on each of the 5-point continua for the eight patient characteristics. Moreover, the patient characteristics appear to be universal—they apply equally well to neonatal, pediatric, and adult patients.

2. The nurse characteristics comprehensively describe the performance level (and competency areas) of nurses who provide direct care to subacute, acute care, and critical care patients. Nurses working with patients at extreme ends of the patient continua identify themselves as having somewhat different levels of competency.

3. The level of patients' needs and the level of nurses' competencies are related; when there is consistency between the patient's characteristics and the nurse's characteristics, optimal outcomes may result. Respondents determined that nurses with higher levels of competency were required to provide direct care to more compromised, critically ill patients.

Discussion and Implications

The current study demonstrated a number of limitations and suggests avenues for further investigation. While few inconsistencies emerged in the data analyses, one inconsistency was noted in regard to the patient profiles: The overall criticality ratings for the adult patient profiles were not linear. That is, nurses ranked the low criticality adult as higher in criticality than the medium criticality adult. Because each profile had been developed by a different SME, and because there are no absolute benchmarks to describe a subacute, acute care, or critical care adult patient, it was not possible to establish a priori control over the acuity level of the profiled patient. Further study, including more comprehensive pilot testing of the patient profiles, should be undertaken to ensure that clear and recognizable differences exist in the status of the patients—independent of the ratings to be assigned by the respondents.

The relationship between nurse self-ratings of their own and their patients' characteristics was somewhat weak. Rater error may have contributed to this finding. There was a ceiling effect in that most respondents self-rated toward the expert end of each rating scale. Observer or supervisor ratings of nurses and their patients might be used to further explore the relationship between patients and nurses.

Even more important, while the results confirmed the expectations inherent in the Synergy Model, simple confirmation falls short of validating the Synergy Model in terms of actually achieving optimal outcomes for patients. Further investigation should be undertaken to determine if nurses who are rated higher on the nurse characteristics actually provide more effective direct care to patients at different levels of need. For example, clinical supervisors might be asked to rate critical care nurses who provide direct care to patients. At the same time, objective measures of optimal outcomes, such as days spent in the unit or the number of rehospitalizations, and patient satisfaction data should be collected and analyzed to determine if differences exist in the course and impact of treatment—that is, in patient outcomes.

Nonetheless, the results were encouraging in suggesting a link between patient needs and required nursing competencies. Based on the results of this research, AACN Certification Corporation adopted the Synergy Model as the guiding framework for its credentialing efforts for critical care nurses and extended the model to describe the nurse characteristics of acute and critical care clinical nurse specialists and progressive care nurses. AACN Certification Corporation currently structures its certification and recertification requirements for critical care nurses, acute and critical care clinical nurse specialists, and progressive care nurses in accordance with the model (Brewer, Wojner-Alexandrov, Triola, Pacini, Cline, Rust, & Kerfoot, 2007).

In the decade since its development, the Synergy Model has been applied to aspects of nursing practice beyond certification. Institutions are using the Synergy Model framework in their nursing practice models. The application of the model to nursing education (Green, 2006; Kaplow, 2003) and the conduct of nursing rounds (Mullen, 2002) have been explored. These applications demonstrate that a highly conceptual and abstract analysis of a profession (i.e., the Synergy Model) can have concrete implications for initial education, certification, and ongoing professional development.

Conceptual Evaluation of the Synergy Model: Process and Results

Karen R. Sechrist, PhD, RN, FAAN
Linda E. Berlin, DrPH, RNC

The AACN Synergy Model for Patient Care™ was developed as a clinical practice model by the American Association of Critical-Care Nurses (AACN) Certification Corporation during a process of reconceptualizing certified nursing practice. Following Synergy Model development and initial testing, the Certification Corporation board of directors (board) identified the need for conceptual evaluation of the Synergy Model by individuals with expertise in nursing theory analysis. The primary goal of the evaluation process was to identify the conceptual strengths and weaknesses of the Synergy Model. A secondary goal was to obtain recommendations regarding refinement of the Synergy Model.

The board contracted with Berlin Sechrist Associates to conduct the evaluation process and appointed a Synergy Model Advisory Group (advisory group) to provide input into all aspects of the process. Members of the advisory group were: Kimmith Jones, MS, RN, CCRN; Aimee Lyons, RN, BSN, CCRN; Patricia McGaffigan, RN, MS, CCRN; and Daphne Stannard, RN, PhD. Martha Curley, RN, PhD, CCRN, was added to the group after selection of the reviewers. Although an overview of the theoretical evaluation process was previously reported (Sechrist, Berlin, & Biel, 2000), a summary of the process is provided as background for the presentation of the findings.

Evaluation Process

The Certification Corporation board was interested in locating nationally known reviewers with significant expertise in analysis of theoretical and conceptual frameworks or models. It was also important to identify reviewers with varying clinical areas of expertise as well as those from varying geographic areas.

Potential reviewers were solicited from among the members of the American Academy of Nurses (AAN). A letter describing the objectives of the evaluation process, the selection criteria for review panel members, and a reprint of Curley's (1998) article "Patient-Nurse Synergy: Optimizing Patients' Outcomes" was sent by mail to all AAN members. Members were invited to self-nominate or encourage non-member colleagues who met criteria to submit applications. A total of 84 individuals responded to the call for reviewers. After review of all credentials, 10 people were recommended to and approved by the advisory group and Certification Corporation board.

Reviewers received a set of all printed materials related to the Synergy Model that were available at the time of the evaluation. The list of printed materials is shown in Figure 15.1.

1. Biel, M. (1997). *Reconceptualizing certified practice: Envisioning critical care practice of the future.* Aliso Viejo, CA: AACN Certification Corporation.
2. *Resource booklet.* (1997). Aliso Viejo, CA: AACN Certification Corporation.
3. Curley, M.A.Q. (1998). Patient-nurse synergy: optimizing patients' outcomes. *American Journal of Critical Care,* 7, 64-72.
4. Edwards, D. F. (1999). The Synergy Model: Linking patient needs to nurse competencies. *Critical Care Nurse,* 19(1): 88-90.
5. Moloney-Harmon, P.A. (1999). The Synergy Model: Contemporary practice of the clinical nurse specialist. *Critical Care Nurse,* 19(2): 101-104.
6. Small, B., & Moynihan, P. (1999). The Synergy Model in practice: The day the lights went out—one charge nurse's nightmare. *Critical Care Nurse,* 19(3): 79-82.
7. Czerwinski, S., Blastic, L., & Rice, B. (1999). The Synergy Model: Building a clinical advancement program. *Critical Care Nurse,* 19(4): 72-77.
8. Biel, M., Eastwood, J. A., Muenzen, P. M., & Greenberg, S. (1999). Evolving trends in critical care nursing practice: results of a certification role delineation study. *American Journal of Critical Care,* 8, 285-290.

Figure 15.1.   List of printed materials about the Synergy Model sent to reviewers.

A form was designed to capture both quantitative and qualitative evaluation information. The form incorporated terminology and essential components for the evaluation of conceptual frameworks or theory from multiple evaluation schema (Barnum, 1998; Fawcett, 1995; Meleis, 1997; Silva & Sorrell, 1992). The final form contained five evaluation criteria: clarity, consistency, adequacy, utility, and significance. Descriptors were identified for each of the evaluation criteria (Table 15.1).

Table 15.1. Synergy Model Evaluation Instrument Criteria, Criterion Descriptors, and Rating Scale Endpoints.

Criteria	Criterion Descriptors	Rating Scale Endpoints
Clarity	• Explanation of the philosophical bases of the Synergy Model • Description of central principle, definitions, and assumptions • Inclusion of meaningful diagrams and explanations • Logic of presentation • Lack of ambiguity • Clarity overall	Unclear to Very Clear
Consistency	• Congruence of model with its philosophical bases • Constancy in use of terms, interpretations and model components • Compatibility of model components • Coherence of model concepts • Consistency overall	Inconsistent to Very Consistent
Adequacy	• Comprehensive of scope within area of concern and level of development • Inclusive of concepts related to person, environment, health, and nursing • Reflective of current nursing realities • Adequacy overall	Inadequate to Adequate
Utility	• Feasibility of using model concepts to guide nursing practice, education, administration, and research • Applicability of the model beyond the critical care setting to other clinical, cultural, and geographic settings • Attainability of projected outcomes • Testability of model concepts • Ability of model to generate quantitative and qualitative research • Utility overall	Not Useful to Useful

Criteria	Criterion Descriptors	Rating Scale Endpoints
Significance	• Delineation of essential issues in nursing • Derivation of nursing interventions influencing patient outcomes • Development of nursing knowledge • Discrimination of nursing from other health professions • Congruence of model with patient, community, and health-care system expectations • Significance overall	Not Significant To Very Significant

Portions of this table appeared in:
Sechrist, K.R., Berlin, L.E., Biel, D.M. (2000). The Synergy Model. Overview of the theoretical review process. *Critical Care Nurse, 20(1),* 85-86.

Reviewers were asked to rate the criterion descriptors within each of the evaluation criteria on a 6-point rating scale, which ranged from total absence of the criterion to absolute presence of the criterion. When descriptors contained more than one item, a rating scale was included for each item. For example, there were three rating scales for the second descriptor under clarity; reviewers were asked to address clarity of the Synergy Model's central principle, definitions, and assumptions.

The rating scale endpoints varied to reflect the evaluation criteria being addressed, as shown in Table 15.1. Space for narrative responses was included along with the rating scale for each of the criterion descriptors. Reviewers were asked to respond to each criterion descriptor to ensure comprehensiveness of responses.

A summary section was included on the review form. Reviewers were asked to address the potential contribution of the Synergy Model to nursing as a discipline, the potential of Synergy Model to positively affect patient outcomes, Synergy Model strengths and weaknesses, and recommendations for Synergy Model refinement.

Review materials and all Synergy Model publications to date were mailed to the reviewers in September 1999. Nine of the 10 reviewers completed the in-depth review process by the November deadline. Members of the Synergy Model Review Panel were: Barbara Stevens Barnum, RN, PhD; Marion E. Broome, RN, PhD, FAAN; Rose E. Constantino, PhD, JD, RN, FAAN, FACFE; Jacqueline Fawcett, PhD, FAAN; Edna M. Menke, PhD, RN; Carolyn Murdaugh, RN, PhD, FAAN; Patricia Moritz, PhD, RN, FAAN; Bonnie Rogers, DrPH, COHN-S, FAAN; and Marilyn Frank-Stromborg, EdD, JD, ANP, FAAN.

Results of the Evaluation

Reviewers provided both quantitative and qualitative evaluation data for criterion descriptors listed under each of the criteria. Rating scale responses for descriptors are presented in tabular form. The total number of responses is less than nine in those instances when one or more of the reviewers chose not to provide a rating for a specific criterion descriptor. Narrative responses were summarized for each descriptor.

Clarity

Rating scale responses for clarity criterion descriptors are shown in Table 15.2. Descriptors with the highest ratings related to the description of the central principle and the logic of Synergy Model presentation. Descriptors with the lowest ratings included those related to meaningful diagrams and lack of ambiguity. A summary of narrative responses follows for each of the clarity criterion descriptors.

Table 15.2. Reviewer Ratings, Means, and Medians for Clarity Criterion Descriptors

| | Ratings | | | | | | | |
| | Unclear | | | | Very Clear | | | |
Criterion Descriptors	1	2	3	4	5	6	Mean	Median
Explanation of philosophical bases (N=9)	2	0	2	1	3	1	3.7	4.0
Description of:								
Central principle (N=9)	1	0	0	3	3	2	4.4	5.0
Definitions (N=9)	1	0	3	4	1	0	3.4	4.0
Assumptions (N=9)	2	0	2	1	2	2	3.8	4.0
Inclusion of meaningful:								
Diagrams (N=9)	1	2	3	2	0	1	3.1	3.0
Explanations (N=9)	0	1	3	4	1	0	3.6	4.0
Logic of presentation (N=9)	0	1	1	1	5	1	4.4	5.0
Lack of ambiguity (N=8)	1	0	2	3	1	1	3.0	4.0
Clarity Overall (N=9)	1	0	1	5	2	0	3.8	4.0

Explanation of the Philosophical Bases of the Synergy Model

Philosophical bases of the Synergy Model were implicit rather than explicit for most reviewers. Two reviewers stated the philosophical bases were clear; two other reviewers found no explanation in the written materials of the philosophical bases or an inconsistent basis. Concerns included: multiple models presented as though they are the same model, inadequate explanation of the decision process to replace past systems with an alternate structure, and lack of discussion of health input-output model variables.

Reviewers suggested making the philosophical basis of the Synergy Model explicit. Specific suggestions included: elaborate on the changes necessitating reconceptualization, clarify the move from implicit to explicit holism if that occurred, clarify the linkages of health systems change to certification, and clarify relationships to other disciplines.

Description of Central Principle, Definitions, and Assumptions

The Synergy Model's central principle and assumptions were clear to most of the reviewers. However, the majority identified a need for additional clarity and consistency of definitions.

Although the central principle of the Synergy Model was clear to most, one reviewer noted that the central principle was stated differently in three of the articles and noted that a clearer statement is needed. The basic premise of "synergy" was problematic for one reviewer because a less critically ill patient requires a less competent nurse. Another reviewer stated that the concept of "safe passage" is not substantiated across documents, and the place of the family in the model needs clarification.

Most reviewers addressed a need for additional clarity and consistency of definitions. A primary area of concern was the lack of definitions, linkages, and clarity in outcomes. The interchangeable use of terms (needs and outcomes, needs and characteristics, characteristics and competencies) also was identified as problematic. General comments from the reviewers were summarized as 1) definitions are not sufficiently descriptive, 2) jargon should be reduced, and 3) descriptions and definitions should be clear enough for the lay public to understand.

Specific comments from individual reviewers were 1) patient characteristics vary in their level of abstraction, 2) nurse characteristics and nurse outcomes are not clear, 3) descriptors for complexity and predictability need clarification, 4) there are ambiguities in leveling (e.g., three levels of outcomes identified), 5) characteristics like clinical judgment need to be defined in other ways than with synonyms, such as clinical reasoning, and 6) synergy needs to be defined more clearly.

Many reviewers indicated the assumptions were clear, and the majority were explicitly stated. One reviewer indicated that the nurse assumptions were sketchy. Another reviewer identified two models, a core model and an outcomes model; the two models were not seen as congruent, and the components were not clear. Specifically, the reviewer indicated that the contribution of "systems" in the core model is unclear, characteristics of nurses are not operationalized in the outcomes model, and it was unclear whether there were seven or eight nurse characteristics.

Inclusion of Meaningful Diagrams and Explanations

Two reviewers indicated that the diagrams and explanations were clear. Other reviewers identified some ambiguity and/or inconsistencies in Synergy Model diagrams and explanations.

There was variation among reviewers regarding the clarity of the diagrams. Two reviewers indicated that the diagrams were clear and helpful. Another reviewer questioned the need for diagrams. Several reviewers indicated that the relationship between patient characteristics, nurse competencies, and outcomes was unclear or implicit, rather than explicit. One additional reviewer indicated that the connections among the three levels of outcomes in the Synergy Model were unclear. Reviewers recommended an additional diagram to clarify the relationship of major Synergy Model concepts/variables.

The "convergence in practice" model was confusing to one reviewer and clearest of all the models to another. One reviewer indicated that the diagrams in the resource booklet were not helpful because of their level of abstraction. Some inconsistencies among diagrams in various publications was noted and attributed to refinements over time. It was suggested by one reviewer that changes be addressed in future publications.

Two reviewers indicated the explanations, for the most part, were clear and expanded on the definitions. One reviewer indicated that explanations for patient characteristics were clear but explanations of nurse characteristics were not as clear. The reviewer noted, further, that the nurse characteristics were not mutually exclusive and the term "collaboration" was used differently by individual authors. Another reviewer stated that the general explanation was clear but how patient characteristics and nurse competencies match and how synergy occurred was ambiguous. The explanation for synergy also was of concern to another reviewer, since it did not seem to explain the process taking place. For this reviewer, "synergy" was viewed as a "holistic term imposed on an essentially logistic system."

Explanations of outcomes and relationships between patient characteristics, nurse competencies, and outcomes were unclear to several reviewers. Additionally, the explanation of "nurse-derived outcomes" was questioned by two reviewers who indicated that outcomes were the result of nursing care rather than nurse outcomes.

A reviewer noted that Synergy Model explanations differed in the various printed materials. The Synergy Model was called a patient-driven model, a nurse-patient relationship model, a patient-nurse-care system model, a patient-family-nurse-care system model, and a model composed of "three spheres of influence"—patient-family, nurse-nurse, and system. These were considered by the reviewer as separate models with different meanings, rather than exemplifying one Synergy Model.

Logic of Presentation

For most reviewers, the logic of the Synergy Model was clear in the presentations. One reviewer noted that assumptions and propositions do not provide a case for nurse outcomes or health systems outcomes. Another suggested identifying how nurses' knowledge and use of assessment related to the Synergy Model. A third reviewer wrote that the authors seemed to address either patient needs or outcomes, rather than both components.

There was a fundamental problem in the logic of the Synergy Model for one reviewer, who noted that synergy is an outcome rather than a process, and that the Synergy Model had no description of what made things happen. Other reviewers also commented that the process was not clear and that the Synergy Model materials did not address how patient characteristics and nurse competencies were linked to produce synergy.

The premise that "patient characteristics drive nurse competencies" was questioned by two reviewers. One reviewer indicated that nurse competencies were developed based on nonpatient experiences in addition to those of the patient. A suggestion was made to define "drive" or select another word. Another reviewer challenged the cause-and-effect relationship in the premise.

Lack of Ambiguity

Most reviewers acknowledged some ambiguity, incompleteness, or inconsistency in the descriptions of the Synergy Model. Several reviewers stated that ambiguity would be expected at the current stage of development and that some ambiguity allowed opportunity for refinement.

An area of ambiguity for several reviewers concerned the linkages among and between patient characteristics, nurse competencies, and outcomes. Other areas of ambiguity included 1) the meaning of synergy and how it occurred, 2) the meaning of caring, 3) definitions and descriptions of outcomes, and 4) inclusion/exclusion of family as a concept. One reviewer suggested testing the assumption that linking patient and nurse characteristics leads to appropriate outcomes. Another indicated that the educational level or background of the nurse needs to be clear.

Clarity Overall

Several reviewers indicated that the philosophical bases of the Synergy Model require clarification. Specifically, they stated that the origins of key concepts were not addressed, there were inconsistencies in perspectives in each paper, and multiple models were presented, rather than one model. One of the reviewers noted that the reasons for reconceptualization were not clear. This reviewer suggested showing how the reconceptualized Synergy Model produced a better fit with holistic models such as those evident in community health.

The meaning of synergy, the causal relationship between patient characteristics and nurse competencies, inclusion or exclusion of the family, and outcomes need to be clarified, according to one or more reviewers. One reviewer indicated that the number of nurse competencies and their definitions require clarification. Descriptions of patient characteristics and the terms, predictability, and complexity were listed as unclear, and it was again noted that some of the diagrams were unclear.

Reviewers addressed lack of clarity in outcomes. Specifically, one or more recommended clarifying the level of outcomes, terms describing the types of outcomes, statements about Synergy Model influences on outcomes, and the relationship of the systems component to outcomes.

Several reviewers noted the clinical and certification relevance of the Synergy Model. One suggested that the Synergy Model has strong points and should be tested. The reviewer indicated that additional evidence is needed for use in certification. Further, use of the term "professional nurse" needs clarification as to whether or not the statement refers to a baccalaureate-prepared RN.

Consistency

Rating scale responses for consistency criterion descriptors are shown in Table 15.3. The mean and median responses for all criterion descriptors are 4.0 or higher. A summary of narrative responses follows for each of the consistency descriptors.

Table 15.3. Reviewer Ratings, Means, and Medians for Consistency Criterion Descriptors.

Criterion Descriptors	Ratings Inconsistent 1	2	3	Consistent 4	5	6	Mean	Median
Model congruence with philosophical bases (N=8)	1	0	1	1	3	2	4.4	5.0
Constancy of:								
Terms (N=9)	0	0	2	2	3	2	4.6	5.0
Interpretation (N=9)	1	0	1	1	3	3	4.6	5.0
Model components (N=9)	2	0	0	1	4	2	4.2	5.0
Compatibility of Model components (N=9)	0	0	0	5	2	2	4.7	4.0
Coherence of Model concepts (N=8)	1	0	0	2	3	2	4.5	5.0
Consistency Overall (N=9)	0	0	1	3	4	1	4.6	5.0

Congruence of the Synergy Model With Its Philosophical Bases

Two reviewers indicated that the Synergy Model was congruent with implied philosophical bases or the Synergy Model's basic premise. Results of the validation study were cited as evidence of congruency by one reviewer. Another reviewer, however, stated that the lack of explicit philosophical bases impacts consistency of the Synergy Model because varying perspectives have resulted.

Two reviewers indicated they could not assess congruence because the philosophical bases were not identified; one suggested that the underlying work of model development still needs to be done. One reviewer noted that ignoring the physiologic elements inherent in critical care produced incongruence, and that the technological role should be addressed to decrease inconsistency. Another reviewer indicated that the arena in which the Synergy Model should function (e.g., critical care or all of nursing) is unclear.

Constancy in Use of Terms, Interpretations, and Synergy Model Components

Most reviewers indicated that terms, interpretations, and Synergy Model components were consistent within and among the materials describing the Synergy Model. Comments follow from those reviewers who identified inconsistencies.

Reviewers identified the following inconsistencies in term use: 1) Patient needs and patient characteristics were used interchangeably; 2) nurse characteristics and nurse competencies were used interchangeably; 3) nurse characteristics included both competencies (clinical judgment, caring behaviors, systems thinking, sensitivity to diversity, clinical inquiry) and roles (advocate, collaborator, evaluator, educator); 4) the number of nurse characteristics varies; and 5) some terms used in the outcomes model were not in the core model. One reviewer asked where clinical skills were located within the characteristics.

A reviewer commented that nursing care results in patient outcomes, and not nurse outcomes, so the use of the term "nurse outcomes" was inconsistent with the literature. The reviewer further indicated that nurse outcomes and nurse-sensitive outcomes were not identical terms.

Interpretation of the Synergy Model within the clinical nurse specialist exemplar program created "fuzziness" for one reviewer. The reviewer also expressed concern that physiologic changes as outcomes were attributed only to nurse influence.

In one of the papers describing the Synergy Model, a reviewer noted that concepts were integrated into another theoretical framework reminiscent of Benner's work. This prompted the reviewer to suggest caution in merging theorists' positions.

An inconsistent interpretation of the Synergy Model's target audience was perceived by one reviewer. The reviewer identified that often the Synergy Model was directed toward critical care nursing, but at other times, the model was directed toward all of nursing.

One reviewer expected both the patient and the family to be major Synergy Model components because one of the articles included both patient and family needs in the title. Another reviewer added that the term "patient" was defined as patient and family, but that the Synergy Model focused on the patient as an individual.

Reviewers stated that the role of outcomes in the Synergy Model was not consistent, because the various models did not all include outcomes. One reviewer expressed uncertainty about the presence of patient and system outcomes and whether family outcomes were included within patient outcomes. Another reviewer identified inconsistent references to the role of the health-care system, since reference to systems included in the article on "safe passage" did not appear in diagrams or definitions of the Synergy Model.

Compatibility of Synergy Model Components

All reviewers acknowledged that the patient characteristics and nurse competencies components of the Synergy Model were compatible; two reviewers cited the validation study as support for compatibility between these Synergy Model concepts. Incompatibilities addressed by reviewers included 1) outcomes not derived from Synergy Model propositions or premises, 2) inconsistencies in discussion of outcomes, and 3) use of the "dialectic" term synergy as either a goal or process, which is inconsistent or incompatible with the "logistic (systems-type) thinking" used to relate patient characteristics and nurse competencies.

Coherence of Synergy Model Concepts

Most reviewers indicated that the Synergy Model concepts were coherent. Two reviewers identified areas of incoherence. One reviewer specified missing connections between patient and nurse characteristics, assumptions about how synergy occurs, and the level of abstraction of concepts as contributors to a lack of coherence. A second reviewer identified several areas contributing to incoherence. They were 1) the context within which the Synergy Model operates varies widely in the various printed materials (see Figure 15.1); 2) synergy, a goal, is used as both a process and a goal; 3) patient needs and patient outcomes are not synonymous, and it is unclear which is the goal; and 4) there are three thought processes evident in the writings (logistic for outcomes, problem-solving for patient needs, and dialectic for synergy). This reviewer further suggested that the concept of synergy is not compatible with systems thinking where specific outcomes are expected.

Consistency Overall

Most reviewers stated that there is consistency in the Synergy Model overall. One reviewer indicated that the Synergy Model is consistent and applicable across nursing specialties. Another reviewer commented that the Synergy Model's internal consistency is intuitive and needs additional testing. A reviewer commented that patient characteristics and nurse competencies "work together" theoretically. Another reviewer added that concepts are philosophically congruent, are related to the literature, and "fit into a structure, process, outcomes framework" logically.

Inconsistencies enumerated by one or more reviewers included 1) conflicting philosophical perspectives; 2) use of the term "patient" to include family at some times and not others; 3) patient characteristics and nurse competencies are used individually at times and as a whole at other times; 4) inclusion of systems components in the outcomes model that do not appear in the core model; 5) multiple models, rather than one Synergy Model; 6) problem with use of the synergy concept with the systems orientation of the Synergy Model; 7) and variations in elements among theory presentations. Recommendations from one reviewer included 1) increasing consistency in references to nurse and patient and patient needs and 2) refinement and clarification of nurse characteristics and levels of outcomes.

Adequacy

Rating scale responses for adequacy criterion descriptors are shown in Table 15.4. Descriptors with the highest ratings included those related to Synergy Model inclusiveness of concepts related to person and nursing. The descriptor with the lowest rating involved Synergy Model inclusiveness of concepts related to environment. A summary of narrative responses follows for each of the adequacy criterion descriptors.

Table 15.4. Reviewer Ratings, Means, and Medians for Adequacy Criterion Descriptors.

| | Ratings | | | | | | | |
| | Inadequate | | | Adequate | | | | |
Criterion Descriptors	1	2	3	4	5	6	Mean	Median
Comprehensive of scope within:								
Area of concern (N=9)	1	0	2	2	3	2	4.0	4.0
Level of development (N=9)	1	0	3	1	4	0	3.8	4.0
Inclusive of concepts related to:								
Person (N=9)	0	0	0	1	6	2	5.1	5.0
Environment (N=9)	2	2	3	1	1	0	2.6	2.5
Health (N=9)	1	0	0	5	3	0	4.0	4.0
Nursing (N=9)	0	0	1	2	5	1	4.7	5.0
Reflective of current nursing realities (N=9)	0	1	3	2	2	1	3.9	4.0
Adequacy Overall (N=9)	1	0	1	4	2	1	4.0	4.0

Comprehensive of Scope Within Area of Concern and Level of Development

There was a diversity of opinion related to comprehensiveness of scope. Several reviewers indicated that the Synergy Model was comprehensive in some areas, but not others.

Most reviewers indicated the Synergy Model was comprehensive. One reviewer indicated that patient characteristics are global and can be applied to all patients.

Several reviewers noted that the Synergy Model is comprehensive in scope in relation to patient and nurse characteristics, but that work remains in the area of outcomes.

Individual reviewers identified limitations of scope in relation to family, community, and nurse-patient interaction.

In terms of level of development, two reviewers indicated that the Synergy Model is at an early developmental stage. One reviewer indicated that scope is difficult to determine because it is unclear for whom the Synergy Model was created. The reviewer suggested continuing developmental work within a critical care context, adding that theories are most applicable within specific specialties. Measurement of Synergy Model variables was addressed by two reviewers who indicated a need for operational definitions and measurement of outcomes.

One reviewer included comments, questions, and suggestions related to the Resource Booklet (see Figure 15.1). Framed as suggestions, they are 1) consider expanding vulnerability descriptors; 2) clarify whether family and friends are included only under the category "social" in Resource Availability; 3) address work impact; 5) consider adding clergy and others to participation in care; 6) include "no desire to participate" under participation in decision-making; 7) address family advocacy under nurse characteristics, advocacy, level 1; 8) include "forward movement" in caring practices in addition to promoting comfort and preventing suffering; 9) address nurse safety; and 10) include aspects of "corporate culture" and change under systems thinking.

Three additional broad suggestions were included by the reviewer. First, additional thought was recommended for the advocacy area in relation to dealing with patient decisions that are not consistent with health, patient actions that can harm self or others, and patient/family disagreement. Second, level I collaboration was perceived as passive, and there was a recommendation to revisit the issue. Third, the reviewer identified an issue of how research conduct should be included and suggested clarification. A second reviewer suggested including statements about the system, environment, and other health-care professionals who collaborate and influence outcomes.

Inclusive of Concepts Related to Person, Environment, Health, and Nursing

Most reviewers perceived that concepts related to person, environment, health, and nursing were included. However, the adequacy of the inclusion varied for the four concepts.

Concepts related to person were identified as clearly present. Several reviewers indicated that "person" in the Synergy Model is the individual patient. One reviewer suggested that "person" be expanded to include family and community; alternately, a rationale should be presented for a more limited view.

Several reviewers stated that a better explanation of environment is needed. One reviewer identified the environment as the nurse-patient relationship, which changed among the various print materials provided for the evaluation process. Most reviewers identified the environment as the critical care or acute care setting, but acknowledged reference to a broader environment in some writings.

Reviewers perceived that health was presented in the context of patient needs. One reviewer indicated that health was described as "ill health," which is consistent with critical care. However, the concept was vague for some reviewers. One reviewer suggested that health was not discussed in terms of a major desired outcome, and that such a discussion would strengthen the outcomes information.

Reviewers indicated that the nursing component related to the competencies of the individual nurse. One reviewer observed that nurse characteristics are "achieved states," while patient characteristics are "inherent states of being." It was noted by another reviewer that a format for nursing process was not explicit.

One reviewer suggested that aggregate level as well as individual level outcomes are important for clinical settings. The reviewer suggested that two Synergy Models may be needed, one for certification in which outcomes are related to the individual nurse, and one that is at an aggregate level with outcomes important to the clinical setting. Another reviewer proposed that comprehensive testing of the Synergy Model be undertaken to identify objective measures of optimal outcomes.

Reflective of Current Nursing Realities

Most reviewers indicated that the Synergy Model is reflective of current nursing realities. Two reviewers indicated that the Synergy Model goes beyond current realities. One reviewer added that the Synergy Model descriptions both reflect and react to current nursing realities. Another reviewer commented that the Synergy Model's complexity reflects the complexity of nursing.

The need for consideration of economic and environmental, system, or contextual influences on nursing practice was addressed by several reviewers. Two reviewers identified the need for testing of the Synergy Model relationships, given current health-care economics.

Adequacy Overall

The majority of reviewers noted that testing is needed to validate adequacy of the Synergy Model. One or two reviewers indicated that 1) the Synergy Model has potential with refinement and testing; 2) the Synergy Model is adequate in some areas but not in all areas (family, outcomes); 3) the scope is adequate for critical care, but additional testing and documentation needs to be completed before suggesting the Synergy Model is useful beyond critical care; and 4) the Synergy Models are worth exploring, but their purposes need to be clarified.

Utility

Rating scale responses for utility criterion descriptors are shown in Table 15.5. Many criterion descriptors had relatively high ratings, including overall utility. There were also several criterion descriptors with relatively low ratings in the areas of geographic applicability, attainability of outcomes, and testability. The number of responses for some of the descriptors was low. Some reviewers indicated the Synergy Model did not provide the needed information or that it was premature in Synergy Model development to evaluate the descriptor. A summary of narrative responses follows for each of the utility criterion descriptors.

Table 15.5. Reviewer Ratings, Means, and Medians for Utility Criterion Descriptors.

| | Ratings | | | | | | | |
| | Not Useful | | | | Useful | | | |
Criterion Descriptors	1	2	3	4	5	6	Mean	Median
Feasibility of using model concepts to guide nursing:								
Practice (N=9)	0	1	0	2	4	3	4.9	5.0
Education (N=8)	1	0	0	1	3	3	4.8	5.0
Administration (N=8)	1	0	0	2	4	1	4.4	5.0
Research (N=8)	0	1	1	1	3	2	4.5	5.0
Model applicability beyond critical care to other settings:								
Clinical (N=7)	0	0	2	1	2	2	4.6	5.0
Cultural (N=7)	1	1	0	3	0	2	3.9	4.0
Geographic (N=7)	1	1	2	0	1	2	3.7	3.0

Criterion Descriptors	Ratings						Mean	Median
	Not Useful			Useful				
	1	2	3	4	5	6		
Attainability of projected outcomes (N=6)	0	0	2	2	2	0	3.9	3.8
Testability of model concepts (N=9)	1	1	3	1	1	2	3.7	3.0
Model ability to generate research:								
Quantitative (N=8)	1	0	0	2	2	3	4.6	5.0
Qualitative (N=8)	0	0	0	3	1	4	5.1	5.5
Utility Overall (N=8)	0	0	0	1	5	2	5.1	5.0

Feasibility of Using Synergy Model Concepts to Guide Nursing Practice, Education, Administration, and Research

All reviewers noted that the Synergy Model has potential use in one or all of the nursing practice, education, administration, and research areas. Most of the reviewers indicated that the Synergy Model has the potential to be feasible for all four areas. Several reviewers stated that Synergy Model use in critical care nursing practice is the most apparent. One reviewer noted that the literature supports use of the Synergy Model to guide practice, but that there are no data to suggest feasibility of use in education, practice, and research. Another reviewer stated that the Synergy Model is an interesting clinical model that needs more development. The reviewer also stated that clinical models do not fit with administration and education and that "no model can do everything." Another reviewer suggested linking the Synergy Model with other relevant models.

Reviewers, for the most part, agreed that the Synergy Model is a feasible guide for nursing practice in critical- and acute-care areas. Several reviewers indicated feasibility for other practice areas as well; two reviewers extended the feasibility to all of nursing. One reviewer indicated high feasibility if administration and education systems were supportive.

Most reviewers stated that it would be feasible to use the Synergy Model for nursing education. Several reviewers perceived that the Synergy Model could be used to assist students in identifying relationships between competency development and meeting patient needs, at least for critical care nursing practice. Ideas expressed by individual reviewers included 1) use of "case scenarios" to aid students in development of nursing characteristics to address differing patient needs and 2) evaluation of students in practicum situations.

Most reviewers stated that it would be feasible to use the Synergy Model for nursing administration. Three reviewers indicated that the Synergy Model might be a guide for staffing and resource allocation decisions. One reviewer suggested that the competency levels might be used as a guide for hiring decisions.

The majority of the reviewers indicated that the Synergy Model can be used to guide nursing research. One reviewer stated that the Synergy Model was too abstract, but that testable propositions could be derived. Two reviewers specifically mentioned the use of the Synergy Model in research on whether certification makes a difference in patient outcomes. One researcher suggested that the current studies should be expanded and continued.

Applicability of the Synergy Model Beyond the Critical Care Setting to Other Clinical, Cultural, and Geographic Settings

Impressions about the applicability of the Synergy Model beyond the critical care setting were mixed. Several reviewers identified broad applicability, while others identified areas requiring developmental work before application. Two reviewers indicated that the literature did not support applicability beyond critical care at this point.

Several reviewers indicated the Synergy Model might be applicable beyond critical care clinical settings, but that the evidence is not there. One reviewer stated that the Synergy Model is applicable in all clinical settings. Another reviewer suggested a clinical area other than critical care in which the Synergy Model could be applicable for certification. One reviewer indicated that the family component in the Synergy Model needs to be expanded for generalization. Two reviewers raised questions about the use of the Synergy Model in healthy populations and primary care.

Reviewers who indicated the Synergy Model is applicable in other cultural settings stated that the Synergy Model is "culturally neutral" or that "cultural utility" is stated in one of the nurse competencies. One reviewer suggested a cultural component be added to the patient characteristics. Two reviewers indicated that assumptions in the Synergy Model related to caring for the sick may differ in other cultures.

To increase usefulness across geographic areas and settings, one reviewer proposed more encompassing definitions of the patient and environment. Another reviewer stated uncertainty regarding Synergy Model usefulness in acute and critical care in rural areas, given the number of nurses available to provide care.

Attainability of Projected Outcomes

Uncertainty of the nature of the projected Synergy Model outcomes was expressed by several reviewers. One reviewer indicated that it was not possible to evaluate attainability from the literature provided for the evaluation process. One reviewer stated that the projected Synergy Model outcomes are difficult to obtain because the Synergy Model is "global and abstract." The reviewer suggested deriving measurable empirical indicators for the outcomes. Most reviewers indicated that significant work needs to be done in this area.

Testability of Synergy Model Concepts

Portions of the Synergy Model were identified by several reviewers as testable once definitions and outcomes are clarified. Three reviewers indicated that the Synergy Model is a grand theory or global conceptual framework that cannot be tested, but can guide the development of testable middle-range theories. One reviewer suggested focusing on the qualitative questions regarding the Synergy Model before proceeding.

Ability of Synergy Model to Generate Quantitative and Qualitative Research

Almost all of the reviewers indicated that the Synergy Model has the potential to generate both quantitative and qualitative research, with the qualification that developmental work remains. One reviewer gave specific examples of research: interaction of patient-nurse characteristics, differentiation of patient and family interactions, outcomes determination, and usefulness of the Synergy Model.

Several reviewers made specific suggestions or cautionary comments regarding use of the Synergy Model in quantitative research. First, reviewers suggested that descriptive quantitative work be undertaken to substantiate the relationships between concepts. One reviewer stated that additional work needs to be done before moving to experimental studies using the Synergy Model as a guide. One reviewer indicated that, while the patient characteristics are the strongest part of the Synergy Model, the use of summative scores is problematic because a total score may inaccurately reflect a significant problem that is out of balance with other problem areas. Also, the divisions in nursing characteristics raise questions if nurses would be ranked.

One reviewer suggested that qualitative research needs to be done to define and describe needs, concepts, and outcomes missing from the Synergy Model. Another suggested that Benner's framework could serve as a typology for work that might occur with the Synergy Model.

Utility Overall

Two reviewers expressed enthusiasm for the Synergy Model. Others indicated it was very feasible with some limitations, including 1) a need for valid and reliable measures; and 2) support from administrators, educators, researchers, and other disciplines. Three reviewers limited the utility to practice, education, and research, while another added administration. One reviewer limited utility to critical care. One reviewer indicated that too little work was done on the Synergy Model to specify its utility.

A reviewer noted the Synergy Model does not have to be perfect to have utility. An additional observation made by the reviewer was that individuals are using parts of the Synergy Model or variations rather than the whole Synergy Model for specific purposes. The fact that it is being used indicated to the reviewer that the Synergy Model deserves further development.

Significance

Rating scale responses for significance criterion descriptors are shown in Table 15.6. Descriptors with the highest ratings involved delineation of essential issues in nursing, development of nursing knowledge, and congruence of the Synergy Model with patient expectations. The descriptor with the lowest rating addressed discrimination of nursing from other health professions. A summary of narrative responses follows for each of the significance criterion descriptors.

Table 15.6. Reviewer Ratings, Means, and Medians for Significance Criterion Descriptors.

| | Ratings | | | | | | | |
| | Not Significant | | | Significant | | | | |
Criterion Descriptors	1	2	3	4	5	6	Mean	Median
Delineation of essential issues in nursing (N=9)	1	0	0	1	4	3	4.8	5.0
Derivation of nursing interventions influencing patient outcomes (N=9)	1	1	2	2	0	3	3.9	4.0
Development of nursing knowledge (N=9)	0	0	1	1	4	3	5.0	5.0
Discrimination of nursing from other health professions (N=8)	0	2	2	3	0	1	3.5	3.5

| | Ratings | | | | | | | |
| | Not Significant | | | Significant | | | | |
Criterion Descriptors	1	2	3	4	5	6	Mean	Median
Congruence of model with expectations:								
Patient (N=8)	0	1	0	1	4	2	4.8	5.0
Community (N=8)	0	2	1	2	2	1	3.9	4.0
Health-care system (N=8)	0	2	0	3	2	1	4.0	4.0
Significance Overall (N=9)	0	1	2	2	1	3	4.3	4.0

Delineation of Essential Issues in Nursing

Several reviewers indicated that the Synergy Model addresses nursing issues. Comments included: provides a guide for "reframing" critical care nursing practice; differentiates levels of care, which may be helpful in resource allocation; may strengthen linkages among practice, education, and research; and addresses nursing competence more thoroughly than elsewhere. One reviewer indicated that nursing issues are not described in the Synergy Model.

The need for outcomes clarity was expressed by three reviewers. One reviewer expressed concern that interest in distancing critical care nursing from medical practice may be detrimental. Another reviewer raised the pragmatic question about the ability of the Synergy Model to work in practice, given current health-care economics. One reviewer suggests that a master's curriculum for acute care should be developed based on the Synergy Model.

Derivation of Nursing Interventions Influencing Patient Outcomes

Variation in responses from reviewers was primarily related to whether interventions were perceived to be immediately derivable or potentially derivable. Comments from those who noted the potential for intervention derivation included: Interventions are implied rather than explicit; the Synergy Model has the potential to be prescriptive and predictive, but is too immature to derive interventions; and nursing competencies are an overview of nursing interventions but are superficial. Suggestions for identification of interventions included: Focus on specific components of the Synergy Model to develop nursing interventions and test their effectiveness; translate competencies into concrete practices carried out by nurses; and consider linking other intervention systems (such as the Iowa Intervention Classification System), if appropriate, to the Synergy Model.

A reviewer commented that specific nursing interventions cannot be derived from the theory elements. The reviewer further suggested that the Synergy Model as presented in the Curley article (see Figure 15.1) presents a logistic, systems model that might be developed to link nursing interventions and patient outcomes.

Development of Nursing Knowledge

Reviewers agreed that the Synergy Model has the potential to contribute to nursing knowledge. Requirements to make that happen were identified as: constructing measures to test the concepts in differing populations, testing (evaluating) the model, and using the Synergy Model as a framework for research. One reviewer indicated the Synergy Model itself is a contribution to nursing knowledge. Another indicated that the Synergy Model clearly goes beyond the function of certification.

Discrimination of Nursing From Other Health Professions

Most reviewers agreed that the Synergy Model does not clearly distinguish nursing from other health professions. One reviewer indicated there is the potential for discrimination and another identified clear distinctions. Two reviewers indicated that the Synergy Model may be useful across professions.

Congruence of Synergy Model With Patient, Community, and Health-Care System Expectations

Most reviewers indicated that the Synergy Model is congruent to some extent with patient and health-care systems expectations, but is less clearly linked to community expectations. One reviewer suggested using the Synergy Model to change expectations.

Two reviewers indicated that patients expect to have their needs addressed, which is congruent with the Synergy Model. Further, patients expect to have a competent nurse and "want the most competent nurse regardless of their level of need."

Synergy Model congruence with community expectations was identified as less clear and dependent on expectations. One reviewer indicated that some of the values, such as quality health care and optimized outcomes, are consistent. Another reviewer noted that the nursing community values the concepts in the Synergy Model, but that students may not be taught to practice in this manner.

Values embraced by health-care systems, such as "cost-effective services, quality patient care, patient satisfaction, and minimal undesirable outcomes" were identified by one reviewer as congruent with the Synergy Model. Another reviewer indicated that the health-care system expectations were reflected in system outcomes. A third reviewer stated that the health-care system relationship is insufficiently addressed. Concerns expressed included the fact that there are few health-care systems that invest in competency development. Another concern listed was the possibility of insufficient "nurse power" to actualize the work as stated in the Synergy Model.

Significance Overall

Three reviewers indicated that the Synergy Model is highly significant. Several others indicated that the potential for significance is present, and that the Synergy Model might have significance beyond critical care.

Individual reviewers commented that the Synergy Model 1) can guide certification and critical care practice that meshes with evolving health-care delivery systems, 2) has the potential to differentiate the impact of nursing care, 3) addresses societal expectations about care and health system needs for controlling cost and optimizing patient outcomes, 4) focuses on the role of the nurse, and 5) has the potential to advance nursing knowledge.

Summary

Reviewers were asked to respond to a set of summary probes. These included:

1. Potential contribution of the Synergy Model to nursing as a discipline.
2. Potential of the Synergy Model to positively affect outcomes.
3. Strengths of the Synergy Model.
4. Weaknesses of the Synergy Model.
5. Recommendations for Synergy Model refinement.
6. Level of theory development.
7. Additional comments.

Responses are presented for each of the summary probes.

Potential Contribution of the Synergy Model to Nursing as a Discipline

Most reviewers indicated that the Synergy Model has the potential to contribute, particularly to the areas of critical care practice and certification, nursing education, and nursing research. Some reviewers stated that the contribution will depend on acceptance in critical-care practice and financial support for continuing Synergy Model development and testing, as well as continuing publications. One reviewer suggested that, once the Synergy Model is refined, a monograph be published that describes the philosophical bases, concepts, relationships, and testing to act as the definitive reference for the Synergy Model. Specific areas identified as needing development included the linkages among patient characteristics, interventions, and outcomes.

One reviewer summarized current contributions to the discipline as follows: 1) identification of patient characteristics and a continuum of needs that is "generalizable across populations," 2) identification of nurse characteristics with the potential for generalizability, 3) descriptions of the interrelatedness of patient needs and nurse competencies that can be tested, 4) a beginning description of patient and system outcomes, and 5) the beginnings of a Synergy Model that may be generalizable.

Potential of the Synergy Model to Positively Affect Outcomes

Most of the reviewers indicated that, if the Synergy Model works in practice, it can positively affect outcomes. One reviewer stated that implementation will be a challenge worth pursuing. Another reviewer was interested in the ability of the Synergy Model to differentiate certified and non-certified nursing practice, particularly if the link to outcomes can be demonstrated.

Discussion of the nature of outcomes was presented by two reviewers. One reviewer recommended reviewing the language of "nurse outcomes," since the context of the patient outcomes was based on nursing care. Further, the reviewer suggested it will be necessary to measure and differentiate both systems outcomes and patient outcomes. Another reviewer stated that the various descriptions of the Synergy Model, other than the Curley description (1998), do not incorporate outcomes and that many of the descriptions confused patient needs and outcomes.

Strengths and Weaknesses of the Synergy Model

Perceptions of Synergy Model strengths and weaknesses are listed in Figure 15.2. One reviewer observed that the narrative accompanying the Synergy Model indicated that development was proactive and designed to enhance clinical care and document practice, as well as demonstrate the importance of nurses. The reviewer also stated that considerable testing remains to be done in critical and acute care.

Synergy Model

Synergy Model Strengths	Synergy Model Weaknesses
• Clear and easy to understand • Logically consistent • Visionary • Parsimonious, including only basic nurse-patient relationship concepts and resulting outcomes • Developed from the evaluation of practice • Reflects current nursing realities • Patient focused; patient characteristics identified and definitions promote operationalization • Exhaustive and mutually exclusive patient characteristics list usable for many purposes • Nursing perspective; nurse competencies identified and definitions developed • Nurse competencies linked to patient outcomes • Inclusion of the health-care system, diversity, consumers in clinical decision-making and collaboration • Potential to test proposed relationships • Potential for use in nursing education, administration, and research • Covers scope of critical-care nursing practice and is generalizable (or potentially generalizable) to all of nursing, all patients and all health-care systems • Feasibility of use at the individual, unit, and organizational level • A beginning restructuring for specialty examinations • Some ambiguity, which allows continuing study and development • Positive energy generated among developers	• Philosophical base(s) not explicit • Origins of key concepts not identified • Concepts and terms not clear and consistent • Patient characteristics or needs • Nurse characteristics or competencies • Ambiguity • How synergy occurs in nurse-patient relationship • Inconsistent use as process and outcome • Inappropriate use as process • Dialectic nature of synergy concept, not synchronous with problematic/systems thinking in the model • Continuum for patient characteristics • Continuum for nurse competencies • Linkages among patient characteristics, nurse competencies, outcomes • Inaccurate statement that patient characteristics "drive" nurse competencies (patient characteristics are not verbs so cannot "drive" nurse competencies) • No consistent model; several models all called Synergy Model • Core model is inconsistent with patient outcomes model • Only the conceptual level of the model described, no explicit relationships • Outcomes component underdeveloped and needs work • Outcomes not addressed in the assumptions or propositions • Outcomes may result from intervening variables not in the model • Individual-focused, but implying system effects • Frequently discussed as though measured at the aggregate level across patients • Role of the family unclear; confounding emphasis on patients and families • Role of the community unclear • Environmental context ignored • No specification of health or nursing process • Rejection of traditional systems approaches without discussion of handling elements in new theory • Negative attitudes toward other health professionals • Implies but does not state that patient acuity and nurse competency should be related, which implies that the most competent nurses should be critical-care nurses • Claims that the model can be used in all areas of nursing practice • Excessive amount of jargon; needs to be understandable to the lay public • Drawings confusing and don't capture interaction

Figure 15.2.   Reviewer perceptions of Synergy Model strengths and weaknesses.

Recommendations for Synergy Model Refinement

Reviewer recommendations for Synergy Model refinement are outlined in Figure 15.3. Reviewer suggestions beyond Synergy Model refinement included 1) development of curricula based on the Synergy Model, 2) reconceptualization and evaluation of the nursing division in several hospitals based on the Synergy Model, and 3) encouragement of doctoral students to develop dissertations based on the Synergy Model. One reviewer expressed interest in seeing papers about the Synergy Model published in non-critical care journals.

1. Decide on the purpose of the model
   a) Ranking of nurses and patients
      i) Develop measurable variables
      ii) Obtain statistical assistance regarding use of rankings
   b) Granting of certification
2. Decide whether the context is critical care or all of nursing
3. Commit to a specific model
   a) Variables unchanging
   b) Definitions unchanging
4. Eliminate the word *synergy* or explain how the model is synergistic
5. Identify origins of key concepts
6. Explicitly describe proposed relationships
   a) Substantiate relationships with available literature to date
   b) Explain how nurse competencies and patient characteristics interact
7. Rework diagrams that depict major components of the model
8. Rework, expand, and make consistent definitions
   a) Patient characteristics
   b) Nurse characteristics
9. Resolve ambiguities
10. Address issues of adequacy
11. Differentiate between patient needs and patient outcomes
    a) Decide which is part of the model
    b) If both kept, identify how each contributes or relates
12. Describe what is meant by the combination of nurse characteristics
13. Rethink outcomes
    a) In terms of three levels of outcomes
    b) In terms of what is meant by nurse-derived outcomes
14. Define, clarify, and test outcomes

15. Develop the systems component in core model
    a) Consider including market demand
16. Clarify the role of family
17. Clarify the role of community
18. Develop mid-range theories to be tested
19. Test the model or components in practice to see if it is pragmatic
20. Continue validation studies

Figure 15.3. Reviewer recommendations for Synergy Model refinement.

Level of Theory Development

Two reviewers indicated that the Synergy Model is a global conceptual model/framework. Another reviewer identified the Synergy Model as a grand theory, less abstract than a conceptual model and more abstract than a middle-range theory. Two reviewers wrote that the focus of future development should be on middle-range or situation-specific theories that can be tested and contribute to knowledge development within the discipline of nursing.

Two reviewers related the level of development to stages of process work by Whitehead or theory development stages from Dickoff and James. For both of these reviewers, the work is at the early stages, with additional attention needed to the hard work of development.

Additional Comments

There were no additional comments related to the conceptual evaluation of the Synergy Model.

The Evaluation Process as an Impetus for Further Work

The overall ratings for each of the criteria are shown together graphically in Figures 15.4 and 15.5. While there was a wide range of opinion among the reviewers related to some of the criteria (see Figure 15.4), the ratings were positive overall.

Ratings and reviewer comments support continued development of the Synergy Model. The reviewers invested significant time and effort in the evaluation process. Their evaluation was thoughtful and their suggestions were reasoned. Comments and suggestions resulting from the evaluation process deserve thoughtful consideration as a basis for further refinement of the Synergy Model by interested individuals and groups.

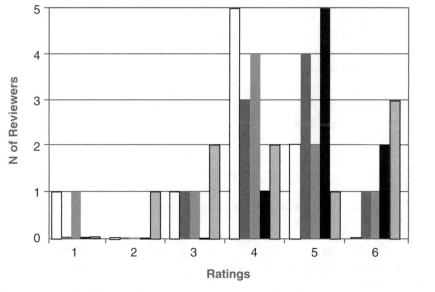

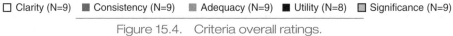

Figure 15.4.   Criteria overall ratings.

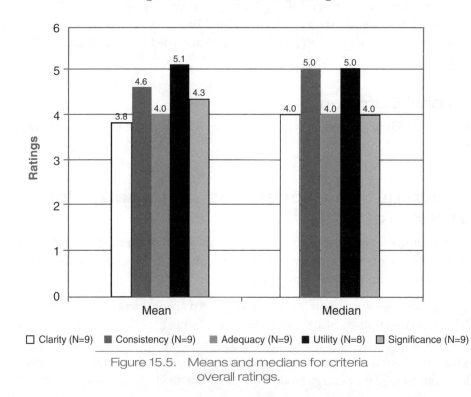

Figure 15.5.   Means and medians for criteria
overall ratings.

Measurement of the Synergy Model

Barbara B. Brewer, PhD, RN, MALS, MBA

"Synergy results when a patient's needs and characteristics are matched with a nurse's competencies" (Curley, 1998, p. 67). Curley's statement is elegant in its simplicity, makes sense to bedside nurses and nurse administrators, and seems pretty straightforward. Yet, implementing the model in practice is not all that simple. Doing so requires measurement of patient needs and characteristics and nurse competencies, and modeling the point at which the two are matched. This chapter will focus on measuring patient characteristics, nurse competencies, and the fit—or synergy—between the two.

Why Measure?

The AACN Synergy Model for Patient Care™ was developed to link nursing practice to patient outcomes (Curley, 1998). The model has been adopted as a framework for academic nursing programs (Zungolo, 2004), clinical education programs (Pacini, 2005), expanding roles of clinical nurse specialists (Cohen, Crego, Cuming, & Smyth, 2002), and as a conceptual model for nursing practice (Kerfoot et al., 2006). The variety of different applications of the model illustrates its broad appeal as a conceptual framework. All of these applications provide some qualitative evidence of the Synergy Model's applicability to nursing, but none of them empirically tests the theoretical relationships specified by the model.

Testing the propositional statements specified in the Synergy Model requires development of operational definitions and empirical indicators of all model variables (Fawcett, 2005). Once definitions and empirical indicators have been specified, the accuracy of statements should be tested through the use of statistical techniques (Walker & Avant, 2005). Testing of the theory in multiple settings with nurses of different experience levels adds credence to the generalizability of the model to different settings. Building sound, comprehensive measures of model variables requires synthesis of the literature regarding each of the model concepts; development of empirical indicators, which are used to observe or measure the phenomenon of interest; and statistical testing to establish reliability and validity of the measures.

Empirical testing of the Synergy Model requires work in the measurement of the nurse competencies, measurement of the patient characteristics, and modeling of the "match" between the two and the relationship of the match to better patient outcomes. To date, case studies have been used to illustrate application of the model in practice, but few studies have actually tested the model in the clinical setting. The case studies are informative, but do not generate knowledge that can be generalized to the population as a whole. The next section will review published work regarding evaluation of nurse competencies.

Nurse Competencies

The Synergy Model specifies eight nurse competencies that are important to patients. The eight competencies include clinical judgment, clinical inquiry, caring practices, response to diversity, advocacy, collaboration, systems thinking, and facilitation of learning (Curley, 1998). Each competency has been defined and is measured along a continuum ranging from novice to expert (see Table 16.1). Most of the literature discussing nurse competencies is descriptive in nature. There are no reports of measuring nurse competency levels in the practice setting. One organization uses these nurse competencies as the framework for differentiating nursing practice in its career advancement program (Kerfoot et al., 2006) and has embedded the nurse competencies in all of its nursing job descriptions and performance appraisals. To date there are no reports in the literature of ties between nurse competencies and patient outcomes.

Table 16.1. Subject Matter Expert Group 5-Point Rating Scale to Anchor the Endpoints and Midpoint of the Continuum Describing Each Nurse Characteristic.

Clinical Judgment

Level 1—Collects basic-level data; follows algorithms, decision trees, and protocols with all populations and is uncomfortable deviating from them; matches formal knowledge with clinical events to make decisions; questions the limits of one's ability to make clinical decisions and delegates the decision-making to other clinicians; includes extraneous detail.

Level 3—Collects and interprets complex patient data; makes clinical judgments based on an immediate grasp of the whole picture for common or routine patient populations; recognizes patterns and trends that may predict the direction of illness; recognizes limits and seeks appropriate help; focuses on key elements of case, while sorting out extraneous details.

Level 5—Synthesizes and interprets multiple, sometimes conflicting, sources of data; makes judgment based on an immediate grasp of the whole picture, unless working with new patient populations; uses past experiences to anticipate problems; helps patient and family see the "big picture"; recognizes the limits of clinical judgment and seeks multidisciplinary collaboration and consultation with comfort; recognizes and responds to the dynamic situation.

Clinical Inquiry

Level 1—Follows standards and guidelines; implements clinical changes and research-based practices developed by others; recognizes the need for further learning to improve patient care; recognizes obvious changing patient situation (e.g., deterioration, crisis); needs and seeks help to identify patient problem.

Level 3—Questions appropriateness of policies and guidelines; questions current practice; seeks advice, resources, or information to improve patient care; begins to compare and contrast possible alternatives.

Level 5—Improves, deviates from, or individualizes standards and guidelines for particular patient situations or populations; questions and/or evaluates current practice based on patients' responses, review of the literature, research, and education/learning; acquires knowledge and skills needed to address questions arising in practice and improve patient care.

Caring Practices

Level 1—Focuses on the usual and customary needs of the patient; no anticipation of future needs; bases care on standards and protocols; maintains a safe physical environment; acknowledges death as a potential outcome.

Level 3—Responds to subtle patient and family changes; engages with the patient as a unique patient in a compassionate manner; recognizes and tailors caring practices to the individuality of patient and family; domesticates the patient's and family's environment; recognizes that death may be an acceptable outcome.

Level 5—Has astute awareness and anticipates patient and family changes and needs; fully engages with and senses how to stand alongside the patient, family, and community; caring practices follow the patient and family lead; anticipates hazards and avoids them, and promotes safety throughout patient's and family's transitions along the health-care continuum; orchestrates the process that ensures patient's/family's comfort and concerns surrounding issues of death and dying are met.

Response to Diversity

Level 1—Assesses cultural diversity; provides care based on own belief system; learns the culture of the health-care environment.

Level 3—Inquires about cultural differences and considers their impact on care; accommodates personal and professional differences in the plan of care; helps patient/family understand the culture of the health-care system.

Level 5—Responds to, anticipates, and integrates cultural differences into patient/family care; appreciates and incorporates differences, including alternative therapies, into care; tailors health-care culture, to the extent possible, to meet the diverse needs and strengths of the patient/family.

Advocacy and Moral Agency

Level 1—Works on behalf of patient; self-assesses personal values; aware of ethical conflicts/issues that may surface in clinical setting; makes ethical/moral decisions based on rules; represents patient when patient cannot represent self; aware of patients' rights.

Level 3—Works on behalf of patient and family; considers patient values and incorporates in care, even when differing from personal values; supports colleagues in ethical and clinical issues; moral decision-making can deviate from rules; demonstrates give and take with patient's family, allowing them to speak/represent themselves when possible; aware of patient and family rights.

Level 5—Works on behalf of patient, family, and community; advocates from patient/family perspective, whether similar to or different from personal values; advocates ethical conflict and issues from patient/family perspective; suspends rules—patient and family drive moral decision-making; empowers the patient and family to speak for/represent themselves; achieves mutuality within patient/professional relationships.

Facilitation of Learning

Level 1—Follows planned educational programs; sees patient/family education as a separate task from delivery of care; provides data without seeking to assess patient's readiness or understanding; has limited knowledge of the totality of the educational needs; focuses on a nurse's perspective; sees the patient as a passive recipient.

Level 3—Adapts planned educational programs; begins to recognize and integrate different ways of teaching into delivery of care; incorporates patient's understanding into practice; sees the overlapping of educational plans from different health-care providers' perspectives; begins to see the patient as having input into goals; begins to see individualism.

Level 5—Creatively modifies or develops patient/family education programs; integrates patient/family education throughout delivery of care; evaluates patient's understanding by observing behavior changes related to learning; is able to collaborate and incorporate all health-care providers' and educational plans into the patient/family educational program; sets patient-driven goals for education; sees patient/family as having choices and consequences that are negotiated in relation to education.

Collaboration

Level 1—Willing to be taught, coached, and/or mentored; participates in team meetings and discussions regarding patient care and/or practice issues; open to various team members' contributions.

Level 3—Seeks opportunities to be taught, coached, and/or mentored; elicits others' advice and perspectives; initiates and participates in team meetings and discussions regarding patient care and/or practice issues; recognizes and suggests various team members' participation.

Level 5—Seeks opportunities to teach, coach, and mentor and to be taught, coached, and mentored; facilitates active involvement and complementary contributions of others in team meetings and discussions regarding patient care and/or practice issues; involves/recruits diverse resources when appropriate to optimize patient outcomes.

Systems Thinking

Level 1—Uses a limited array of strategies; limited outlook—sees the pieces or components; does not recognize negotiation as an alternative; sees patient and family within the isolated environment of the unit; sees self as key resource.

Level 3—Develops strategies based on needs and strengths of patient/ family; able to make connections within components; sees opportunity to negotiate but may not have strategies; developing a view of the patient/ family transition process; recognizes how to obtain resources beyond self.

Level 5—Develops, integrates, and applies a variety of strategies that are driven by the needs and strengths of the patient/family; global or holistic outlook—sees the whole rather than the pieces; knows when and how to negotiate and navigate through the system on behalf of patients and families; anticipates needs of patients and families as they move through the health-care system; utilizes untapped and alternative resources as necessary.

As discussed in chapter 14, a tool was developed to evaluate expertise in each of the nurse competencies. The tool includes a definition and a 5-point rating scale, with behavioral anchors illustrating novice, intermediate, and expert practice on each of the eight competencies. In their three-part study, they asked nurses to rate the proportion of their own patients at each point on the patient characteristics scale, rate their own performance on the nurse competencies scale, and then rate the criticality of three hypothetical patients on a low, medium, or high scale. They also ranked the same three hypothetical patients using the patient characteristics scale and indicated the level of competency required to achieve optimal outcomes for each of the patients. The researchers reasoned that nurses would identify higher levels of competency as necessary to care for more compromised patients. This last part of the study was intended to evaluate the model tenet that the match between patient needs and nurse competencies would result in optimal patient outcomes.

The nurse competencies measure performed as expected. Nurses who had greater levels of experience rated themselves higher on the continuum for each of the eight nurse competencies. Cohen, Crego, Cuming, and Smyth (2002) translated the eight nurse competencies into clinical nurse specialist (CNS) practice. They described how CNSs facilitate competencies in staff nurses or use them to shape their own practices. For example, CNSs served as role models in clinical inquiry by actively participating in development of evidence-based policies and procedures, critiquing and sharing research articles with staff nurses, becoming members of an institutional review board, and presenting research topics. The authors provided examples or case studies for all eight competencies. They suggested that incorporating the Synergy Model into their practice resulted in better patient outcomes, but they did not provide any evidence to support their claim.

Much of the literature regarding application of nurse competencies involves case studies or descriptions of methods of model application. None of the reports in the literature quantify nurse competencies in the practice setting.

Patient Characteristics

The Synergy Model specifies eight patient characteristics that are important to nurses. The eight patient characteristics are stability, complexity, predictability, resiliency, vulnerability, participation in decision-making, participation in care, and resource availability (Curley, 1998). Patient characteristics should drive patient care assignments of nurses and should be based on matching patient needs with nurse competencies. There are several reports in the literature of studies measuring patient characteristics in the acute-care setting.

As part of the validation study described in Chapter 14, Greenberg, Muenzen, and Smith developed a measure of patient characteristics. Subject matter experts were used to define each patient characteristic and a rating scale containing a single 5-point indicator for each characteristic (see Table 16.2). Lower scores indicate greater criticality. For example, a score of one on the complexity indicator reflects a patient who has an intricate or atypical presentation, while a score of five reflects a patient who has a routine, fairly straightforward presentation. Findings from their study supported the criticality of the patient characteristics measure—that is, nurses who worked in critical care units rated their patients on the more compromised end of the patient characteristics scale than did nurses who worked in acute and ambulatory care. The authors also reported that there was a strong relationship between patient acuity and six of the eight patient characteristics (stability, complexity, predictability, resiliency, vulnerability, and participation in care). Nurses' ratings of their patients' characteristics reflected patients they had cared for during the previous month.

Table 16.2. Subject Matter Expert Group 5-Point Rating Scale to Anchor the Endpoints and Midpoint of the Continuum Describing Each Patient Characteristic.

Stability

Level 1—Minimally stable—Labile; unstable; unresponsive to therapies; high risk of death.

Level 3—Moderately stable—Able to maintain steady state for limited period of time; some responsiveness to therapies.

Level 5—Highly stable—Constant; responsive to therapies; low risk of death.

Complexity

Level 1—Highly complex—Intricate; complex patient/family dynamics; ambiguous/vague; atypical presentation.

Level 3—Moderately complex—Moderately involved patient/family dynamics.

Level 5—Minimally complex—Straightforward; routine patient/family dynamics; simple/clear-cut; typical presentation.

Predictability

Level 1—Not predictable—Uncertain; uncommon patient population/illness; unusual or unexpected course; does not follow critical pathway, or no critical pathway developed.

Level 3—Moderately predictable—Wavering; occasionally noted patient population/illness.

Level 5—Highly predictable—Certain; common patient population/illness; usual and expected course; follows critical pathway.

Resiliency

Level 1—Minimally resilient—Unable to mount a response; failure of compensatory/coping mechanisms; minimal reserves; brittle.

Level 3—Moderately resilient—Able to mount a moderate response; able to initiate some degree of compensation; moderate reserves.

Level 5—Highly resilient—Able to mount and maintain a response; intact compensatory/coping mechanisms; strong reserves; endurance.

Vulnerability

Level 1—Highly vulnerable—Susceptible; unprotected, fragile.

Level 3—Moderately vulnerable—Somewhat susceptible; somewhat protected.

Level 5—Minimally vulnerable—Safe; out of the woods; protected, not fragile.

Participation in decision making

Level 1—No participation—Patient and family have no capacity for decision-making; require surrogacy.

Level 3—Moderate level of participation—Patient and family have limited capacity; seek input/advice from others in decision-making.

Level 5—Full participation—Patient and family have capacity and make decisions for themselves.

Participation in care

Level 1—No participation—Patient and family unable or unwilling to participate in care.

Level 3—Moderate level of participation—Patient and family need assistance in care.

Level 5—Full participation—Patient and family fully able to participate in care.

Resource availability

Level 1—Few resources—Necessary knowledge and skills not available; necessary financial support not available; minimal personal/psychological supportive resources; few social systems resources.

Level 3—Moderate resources—Limited knowledge and skills available; limited financial support available; limited personal/psychological supportive resources; limited social systems resources.

Level 5—Many resources—Extensive knowledge and skills available and accessible; financial resources readily available; strong personal/psychological supportive resources; strong social systems resources.

Other findings supportive of validity of the patient-characteristics measure reported by the researchers were inter-item correlations among the patient-characteristics indicators and the results of exploratory factor analysis. Exploratory factor analysis was performed for adult, pediatric, and neonate age groups. Each resulted in a two-factor solution, but there were differences in factor loadings among the three groups. Data from nurses who cared for pediatric and neonatal patients resulted in stability, complexity, predictability, resiliency, and vulnerability, loading on the first factor, while participation in decision-making, participation in care, and resource availability loaded on the second factor. In the analysis performed on data from nurses caring for adult patients, loadings on the first factor were similar, except predictability loaded with items in the second factor. The authors suggested that the first factor reflects characteristics intrinsic to the individual patient and family, and the second factor reflects characteristics that are extrinsic.

Brewer and colleagues (Brewer, Pacini, Triola, Wallace, & Wojner-Alexandrov, 2005; Brewer, Wojner-Alexandrov, Triola, Pacini, Cline, Rust et al., 2007) reported a study testing the reliability and validity of the patient characteristics measure in a three-hospital tertiary care system. The study was done in two phases. Phase one was a study evaluating reliability and validity of the patient characteristics measure in a sample of patient ratings done by nurses expert in the Synergy Model (N=481); phase two involved reliability and validity evaluation in a sample of patient ratings completed by nurses who had not been previously exposed (naïve nurses) to the Synergy Model (N=279). Internal consistency reliability was acceptable in both samples (Chronbach's alpha = .88 in both studies). Construct validity was evaluated using exploratory factor analysis and known-group validity.

Inter-item correlation coefficients were similar to those found by Greenberg, Muenzen, and Smith (see chapter 14) and ranged from r=.22 to r=.75 in the expert group and r=.29 to r=.78 in the naïve nurse group. Exploratory factor analysis was performed using principal components extraction with varimax rotation. The resulting two-factor solution was similar to that found by Greenberg, Muenzen, and Smith, except in both phases of the study done by Brewer and colleagues (2005, 2007), items loaded consistently on the same factor. The researchers identified the first factor as one containing the patient's intrapersonal characteristics (stability, complexity, resiliency, predictability and vulnerability) and the second factor as one containing the patient's interpersonal characteristics.

The second measure of construct validity, differences among known groups, performed differently in the two samples. In their study, Brewer and colleagues (2005, 2007) split the sample into three groups based on patient acuity unit type, critical care, acuity adaptable (universal), or general care. In all cases in the expert nurse group, patients who were located in critical care units had statistically lower patient characteristics scores than did patients located in the other two unit types. This was not the case in the naïve nurse sample, where differences were found in only three of the eight patient characteristics: resiliency, vulnerability, and participation in care. This finding was of concern and requires further research to evaluate the measure in a general population of nurses.

A third study evaluating the ability of a patient classification tool to act as a proxy for the patient-characteristics measure was reported by Brewer (2006). In this study, the researcher created multilevel variables from dichotomous workload indicators of a proprietary patient classification system. The new variables were created to facilitate evaluation of linear relationships among the eight Synergy patient characteristics variables and the acuity scores. Brewer reported small relationships among the acuity items and the patient characteristics variables except for participation in care, which exhibited moderate relationships with six acuity indicators, activities of daily living, activities of daily living with the support of two people, fluid management, skin care, pulmonary management, and cardiovascular/neurological management. She suggested that acuity indicators were not good substitutes for patient characteristics.

Measurement Issues

When developing a new scale, it is best to ground the scale in substantive theory related to the phenomenon of interest (DeVellis, 1991). Greenberg, Muenzen, and Smith report that subject matter experts were used to develop the scale items for both the patient characteristics and nurse competency measures. What is not clear is whether thorough concept analyses were performed for each of the eight characteristics represented by the patient measure. Concept analyses would aid in the development of domains for each of the characteristics constructs. Once the domains are specified, items could be generated that adequately tap into each domain. Single item scales for each of the eight patient characteristics may not adequately measure the phenomena of interest.

McIver and Carmines (1981) suggest that multiple items are better than single-item, one-dimensional scales for several reasons, including the inability of a single item to capture complex theoretical concepts, lack of precision, proneness to random error, and lack of sufficient information to evaluate measurement properties. The patient characteristics measure consists of eight items representing eight different one-dimensional scales, rather than a single one-dimensional scale with multiple (eight) items.

In its current format, each patient characteristics item consists of scale anchors containing several adjectives attempting to capture the multiple attributes of its respective concept. Based on the suggestion of McIver and Carmines (1981), revising the scale to include a single item for each adjective pair would strengthen its measurement properties by reducing random error and increasing precision regarding the level of each attribute. For example, the adjectives for level one complexity (highly complex patients) are intricate, complex patient/family dynamics, atypical, ambiguous/vague. It would be highly unusual for a single patient to score level one for each of the conditions/situations specified under the level one option. What if the patient was a one on all but family dynamics, which were routine? How would a nurse be expected to score that patient? Would she give the patient three 1s and a 5 for an average score of 2? Would the patient receive a different rating if each of the four options were separate items? Would separate items increase the ability of the scale to show variability among patients? Improving the ability of the measure to discriminate among subtle differences would maximize variability and improve its ability to correlate with other measures (DeVellis, 1991). Improving the ability of each variable to correlate with other measures is vital for model testing.

Another problem related to the adjective anchors is that the number of adjectives is inconsistent at each end and in the middle of the indicators. For example, the vulnerability indicator includes three adjectives describing the level one option (susceptible, unprotected, fragile), two adjectives describing the level three option (somewhat susceptible, somewhat protected), and four adjectives describing the level five option (safe, out of the woods, protected, not fragile). Does the imbalance in the number of adjectives affect ratings? Is the rater able to clearly distinguish between a level one, level three, or level five patient on this characteristic? How much random error does the imbalance introduce?

Other issues with the scale involve the clarity and comprehensiveness of the individual items. Brewer (2006) reports that some of the nurses who completed ratings had difficulty with the stability item. Some nurses in her study thought that the item referred to balance (stability on their feet) versus hemodynamic equilibrium. DeVellis (1991) suggests that item characteristics that consistently separate good scale items from not-so-good scale items are related to clarity. Ambiguity of statements will lead to measurement error from differences in interpretation by individuals completing the scale. For example, the stability indicator definition is "the ability to maintain a steady-state equilibrium" (Curley, 1998). Response choice adjectives for this item include unresponsive to therapies, unstable, labile, and at high risk of death. One can see how a nurse who cares for patients on an orthopedic unit may have a different interpretation of stability from one who works with cardiovas-cular patients. An orthopedic nurse may interpret unresponsive to therapies as lack of physical gains from physical therapy, while a cardiovascular nurse may interpret the same statement as lack of hemodynamic response to sympathomimetic drug therapy. A good scale should be able to discriminate between these two very different situations; otherwise, it may be too ambiguous and should be revised.

Stability

Research needs to be conducted to establish the stability of the items. To date there have been no reports of studies evaluating test-retest reliability. As a result, it is unknown if the measure performs consistently over time. In addition, if the measure is to be used in prac-tice, theoretical stability of each patient characteristic must be established. Some patient characteristics may require ratings every shift, others may require ratings when levels of care are changed (critical care to medical-surgical and vice-versa), while others may re-quire ratings once during a hospital stay. For example, over what interval of time would we expect vulnerability to be consistent in an individual patient? Would we expect the level of vulnerability to be the same over an 8-hour period, a 12-hour shift, a day, at each level of care, or throughout an entire hospital stay? Does the interval differ by characteristic? For example, would we expect resource availability to vary from shift to shift or day to day? Would resource availability be consistent throughout an entire hospital stay? These are im-portant questions, because their answers affect the frequency required for accurate ratings, as well as help us understand the required measurement burden placed on the nursing staff.

Synergy: Testing the Match

The final section of this chapter will address measuring synergy, or the fit, between nurse competencies and patient characteristics. The model specifies that different nurse competencies are required for different levels of patient characteristics. In other words, the types and amounts of nurse competencies depend on the types of patients typically managed on a unit. The model further specifies that once the match between the two is made, the patient will achieve optimal outcomes and safe passage through the hospital stay.

In the practice validation study cited above, Greenberg, Muenzen, and Smith found support for the linkage between nurse competencies and patient characteristics, and then surmised that consistency between the two may result in optimal patient outcomes. Nurses were asked to rate three hypothetical patients on their level of patient characteristics and criticality. Then they were asked to rate the level of nurse competencies required for each of the three patients. The researchers reported that patient characteristics correlated with nurse competencies in all hypothetical patients, but were weaker in the hypothetical adult patient than the pediatric or neonate.

To date, no one has empirically tested the conceptual linkages between nurse competencies and patient characteristics with actual patients, or linked the relationship between nurses and patients with outcomes. Measurement of the match between nurses and patients against optimal outcomes requires that we use regression analysis to test the effect of the combination of patient characteristics and nurse competencies on different patient outcomes (Schoonhoven, 1981). The selection of outcomes may be determined by the population or types of patients typically managed on a patient care unit or within a hospital. Research is needed in this area to establish linkages, which can then be translated into the clinical setting.

Testing cannot be undertaken without first resolving measurement issues identified with the patient characteristics scale and establishing satisfactory measurement properties of the nurse competency scales. Once the best combination of nurses with patients is established, the information may be used to make important hiring considerations about nurses, as well as to make daily patient care assignments. Profiles regarding the number and type of each competency needed to optimize patient care for a unit could be established. Outcomes over time for patients cared for on these units could then be evaluated to test the effectiveness of the match. Outcome measurement must include contextual variables to account for differences in patient care environments. The information from this type of research may possibly be used to formulate dose-response curves suggested by Titler (2004).

Summary

The Synergy Model has been adapted in multiple settings despite limited empirical support for the model's tenets. Scale development based on sound concept analyses for each of the eight nurse competencies and eight patient characteristics should be considered. Once sound measures are established, the match between the two may be tested to evaluate relationships with patient outcomes. Results of empirical studies can be used to develop staffing profiles for different patient unit types, which will support adoption of the model in clinical practice.

How the Synergy Model Was Developed

Martha A.Q. Curley, RN, PhD, FAAN

In 1992, the board of directors of the American Association of Critical-Care Nurses (AACN) Certification Corporation (see Table A.1) initiated discussions regarding the need for a new conceptual model that better described CCRN[1] certified practice. This was necessary because the AACN Certification Corporation was planning its third role-delineation study to assure the CCRN test blueprint reflected contemporary critical care nursing practice (Niebuhr, 1993). At that time, the CCRN designation was held by more than 50,000 critical care nurses, and the link among certification, practice, education, and improved patient outcomes was difficult to describe. The board of directors noted that a major change in thinking about certified practice was required. The CCRN exam blueprint needed to shift from a body-system disease framework to a more holistic model that articulated both the art and science of contemporary critical care nursing practice.

---

[1]CCRN® is a registered service mark of the AACN Certification Corporation and denotes certification in critical care nursing as granted by the AACN Certification Corporation.

Table A.1. 1992 AACN Certification Corporation Board of Directors

Gayle R. Whitman, RN, MSN, FAAN (Chair)

Mickey Stanley, RN, PhD, CCRN (Chair-Elect)

Claire E. Sommargren, RN, BSN, CCRN (Secretary/Treasurer)

Robert A. Murphy (Consumer Representative)

Karen K. Carlson, RN, MN, CCRN

Martha A.Q. Curley, RN, MSN, CCRN

Cindy Strzelecki, RN, BSN, CCRN

Staff:

Sarah Sanford, RN, MA, CNAA, FAAN (CEO)

Bonnie McCandless, RN, MS (Director of Certification)

One of the first activities of the newly designated AACN Certification Corporation board was to build consensus around a vision that would help guide certification activities. The board envisioned "Critical care practice driven by patient needs which directly contributes to optimal patient outcomes." The AACN Certification Corporation board vision, which focused on nursing practice, complemented its membership's vision, "A health-care system, driven by the needs of patients, in which critical care nurses make their optimal contribution," which focused on the health-care system.

In June 1993, Gayle R. Whitman, chair of The AACN Certification Corporation board, convened a think tank (see Table A.2) to develop a conceptual model that would link the certification program to its new vision; specifically, to identify dimensions of certified practice that were most likely to meet patient needs and contribute to optimal patient outcomes.

Table A.2. Think Tank Members

Martha A.Q. Curley, RN, MSN, CCRN

Mairead Hickey, RN, PhD

Pat Hooper, RN, MSN, CCRN (Kyriakidis)

Wanda Roberts Johanson, RN, MN

Bonnie Niebuhr, RN, MS (McCandless)

Sarah Sanford, RN, MA, CNAA, FAAN

Gayle R. Whitman, RN, MSN, FAAN

The think tank met twice in Boston, Massachusetts: September 8-9, 1993, and March 25-24, 1994. During this second meeting, the think tank reached agreement on the fundamental aspect of the evolving conceptual model—specifically, that patient needs or characteristics drive and determine nurses' competencies (AACN Certification Coporation, 1995). The think tank identified 13 preliminary patient characteristics, including patient compensation, resiliency, margin of error, predictability, complexity, vulnerability, physiological stability, risk of death, independence, self-determination, involvement in care decisions, engagement, and resource availability. The group acknowledged the overlap between these patient dimensions but recommended that a separate subject matter expert (SME) group (See Table A.3) be formed to operationally define each dimension and modify as necessary.

Table A.3. Study of Practice Subject Matter Experts

Martha A.Q. Curley, RN, MSN, CCRN
DuAnne Foster-Smith, RN, MN, CCRN
Janet Fraser Hale, RN, CS, PhD, CCR, FNP
Deborah Gloskey, RN, MS, CCRN
Teresa Halloran, RN, MSN, CCRN
Sonya Hardin, RN, PhD, CCRN
Mairead Hickey, RN, PhD
Patricia Hooper, RN, PhD
Vicki Keough, RN, MSN, TNS, TNCC
Patricia Moloney-Harmon, RN, MS, CCRN
Kathleen Shurpin, RN, PhD, CS, ANP, OCN
Daphne Stannard, RN, MS, CCRN

Staff:
Melissa Biel, RN, MSN (Staff, AACN Certification Corporation)
Sandy Greenberg, PhD (PES)
Pat Muenzen, MA (PES)
Leon Smith, PhD (PES)

The think tank noted that each patient dimension addressed the whole person (body, mind, spirit) in health and illness. Thus, each patient dimension was dynamic and could be defined along a continuum—for example, of low risk for death to high risk for death.

The think tank also initially identified nine dimensions of nursing practice required to meet the identified patient needs. These included engagement, skilled clinical practice, agency, caring practices, systems management, teamwork, diversity responsiveness, experiential learning, and innovator/evaluator. The group again acknowledged the potential overlap between the nurse dimensions and again recommended that an SME group meet to operationally define each dimension and modify as necessary.

The nursing practice dimensions were also described along continuums driven by the needs of patients, each reflecting a dynamic integration of knowledge, experience, and skill. The think tank noted that in certified practice, a dynamic interaction exists between patient needs and nurse competencies. Patient needs and nurse competencies synthesize in a circular fashion by which nurse-patient interaction influences patient needs, which in turn influence the next nurse-patient interaction. The relationship continues until the end-point is reached—specifically, when the needs of the patient are optimally met.

In March 1995, the AACN Certification Corporation board joined with Professional Examination Service (PES) to conduct a Study of Practice. The Study of Practice approach was different than past role-delineation studies that focused on existing job tasks and knowledge. The Study of Practice SME was charged with establishing nursing characteristics required to meet patients' needs currently and in the future. The SME would refine and validate the patient-driven "synthesis" model, examine dimensions of certified practice that were required to meet patients' needs and contribute to optimal patient outcomes, and reorient how nursing practice was defined.

The SME group met June 9-11, 1995, in Chicago and October 21-23 of that year in Boston. The group worked to describe patients of all ages across the widest range of practice settings. Operational definitions and a continuum of descriptors were developed and then refined for each patient characteristic (see Table A.4) and nurse characteristic (see Table A1-5). Each continuum was critically evaluated for potential omission and overlap. Several continua—specifically, compensation, margin of error, risk of death, independence, engagement, and experiential learning—were eliminated because of redundancy. Preliminary assumptions of the model were identified. These included:

1. The whole person is considered: body, mind, spirit.

2. The context in which the nurse-patient interaction occurs impacts each dimension. Consideration is given to the patient/family/community biological, psychological, social, and spiritual dynamic as well and the patient/family/community's developmental stage.

3. The dimensions are not independent and cannot be considered in isolation. All are considered collectively to ascertain a quantifiable profile of the patient. This is also true of the nurse dimensions.

4. The goal of nursing is to restore the patient to an optimal level of wellness as defined by the patient and family. Death can be an acceptable outcome, in which the goal of nursing care is to move the patient toward a peaceful death.

Table A.4.   Patient Characteristics

(Extrapolated from August 1995, October 1995, and March 1996 SME minutes)

1. Stability: The ability to maintain a steady state.

   Stable (physiological, emotional, social, spiritual)

   - Effective compensation and coping
   - Constant state
   - Responsive to therapy
   - Low risk of death

   Unstable

   - Ineffective compensation
   - Labile state
   - Unresponsive to therapy
   - High risk of death

2. Complexity: The intricate entanglement of two or more systems.

   Simple

   - Routine case
   - Straightforward
   - Single organ dysfunction
   - No comorbid condition
   - Routine family dynamics

   Complex

   - Complicated case
   - Multiproblem disorder
   - Multisystem condition
   - Complex family dynamics

3. Vulnerability: Susceptibility to stressors that may adversely affect patient outcomes.

   Minimally vulnerable

   - Safe/protected
   - Minimal risk
   - Impervious

   Vulnerable

   - Not safe/unprotected
   - Open to threat
   - "At risk"
   - Potentially compromised
   - Easily influenced
   - Susceptible

4. Predictability: A characteristic that allows one to expect a certain trajectory of illness.

   Predictable
   - Certain
   - Routine
   - Expected response
   - Common patient population/illness

   Unpredictable
   - Uncertain
   - Unexpected response
   - Uncommon patient population/illness

5. Resiliency: The capacity to return to a restorative level of functioning using compensatory mechanisms.

   Resilient
   - Strong reserves
   - Returns to individual baseline rapidly
   - "Bounce back"
   - Hardiness
   - Survivor
   - Tolerant

   Minimally resilient
   - Limited reserve
   - Returns to individual baseline slowly
   - No bounce
   - Fragile
   - Intolerant

6. Participation in decision-making: Extent to which the patient engages in decision-making.

   Engaged
   - Independent
   - Autonomous
   - Capacity for self-determination
   - Able

   Minimal engagement
   - Decision-making completely guided by others
   - Dependent on others
   - Incapable or lacks capacity to engage

7. Participation in Care: Extent to which the patient participates in care.

   Participates in Care
   - Capable
   - Involved
   - Engaged

Minimal participation in care

- Unwilling or unable to care for self
- Not involved
- Care determined by others
- Not engaged

8. Resource Availability: Extent of resources the patient/family/community bring to the care situation.

Adequate

- Insured
- Strong social support
- Multiple caregivers
- Adequate knowledge and skill
- Plentiful equipment

Inadequate

- Not insured
- Few or no social supports
- Few or no caregivers
- Inadequate knowledge and skill
- Equipment in short supply

Table A.5 Nurse Competencies.

The left column reflects competent nursing practice. The right column reflects expert nursing practice.

(Extrapolated from August 1995, October 1995, and March 1996 SME minutes)

---

1. **Clinical Judgment: Clinical reasoning, which includes clinical decision-making, critical thinking, and a global grasp of the situation, coupled with nursing skills acquired through a process of integrating formal and experiential knowledge.**

• Collects basic level data.	• Synthesizes and interprets multiple, sometimes conflicting, sources of data (e.g., honing in on key elements while sorting our extraneous detail).
• Uncomfortable deviating from algorithms, decision trees, and protocols.	
• Matches formal knowledge with clinical events to make decisions.	• Makes judgments based on an immediate grasp of the whole clinical picture; uses past experiences to anticipate problems.
• Questions the limits of one's ability to make clinical judgments and delegates decision-making to other clinicians.	• Recognizes patterns and trends that situate patients in a trajectory.
• Concerned about issues related to the patient on one's shift.	• Recognizes the limits of one's clinical judgment and is comfortable seeking multidisciplinary collaboration or consultation.
	• Responsive to the dynamic situation.
	• Helps the patient and family see big picture.

2. **Clinical Inquiry: The ongoing process of questioning and evaluating practice and providing informed practice. Creating practice changes or innovation through research utilization and experiential learning.**

- Begins to question practice and compares and contrasts possible alternatives
- Implements changes in practice developed by others
- Provides cost-effective care
- Understands the scientific basis for actions

- Individualizes guidelines for particular patients
- Evaluates and innovates practice
- Challenges the status quo
- Builds a case for change and acts on data
- Active role in solving problems

Clinical judgment and inquiry converge at the expert level

3. **Caring practices: The constellation of nursing activities that are responsive to the uniqueness of the patient and family and that create a compassionate and therapeutic environment with the aim of promoting comfort and preventing suffering. These caring behaviors include, but are not limited to, vigilance, engagement and responsiveness.**

- Attentive to the usual and customary needs of the patient and family
- Watchful
- Maintains a safe humanistic environment
- Engages patient and family in a compassionate manner

- Astute awareness to the subtleties of suffering
- Vigilant – uses self as monitor
- Follows the patient's or family's lead
- Presence (empathy, warmth)
- Fully engaged with and senses how to stand alongside the patient and family
- Preserves life world
- Orchestrates a process that ensures the patient's/family's comfort and concerns surrounding death and dying are met

4. **Response to Diversity: The sensitivity to recognize, appreciate and incorporate difference into the provision of care.**
Differences may include, but are not limited to individuality, cultural differences, spiritual beliefs, gender, racial, ethnicity, family configuration lifestyle, socioeconomic status, age, values, alternative medicine involving patients/families and members of the health-care team.

- Recognizes personal bias
- Inquires about differences and considers their impact on care
- Accommodates personal and professional differences in the plan of care

- Appreciates and incorporates differences into care
- Values personal and professional differences

- Demonstrates tolerance
- Accepting of differences
- Helps the patient and family understand the culture of the health-care system
- Aware of roles of members of health-care teams

- Tailors the health-care culture to meet the diverse needs and strengths of the patient and family

5. **Advocacy/moral agency: Working on another's behalf and representing the concerns of the patient/family/community. Serves as a moral agent in identifying and helping to resolve ethical and clinical concerns within the clinical setting.**

- Beginning advocacy (works on behalf of patients)
- Aware of one's own personal values
- Aware of ethical conflicts that occur in one's clinical setting; makes ethical decisions based on rules
- Aware of patient and family rights
- Accountable for one's own practice
- Respects patient and family
- Represents patient when patient cannot represent self

- Anticipates and assumes a leadership role in resolving ethical conflict
- Agent—gives voice to patients; serves as an instrument
- Suspends rules; patient and family drive ethical decision-making
- Empowers the patient and family to speak for themselves
- Achieves mutuality within patient/professional relationships
- Values differences

6. **Facilitator of learning: The ability to use self to facilitate learning**

- Follows a planned educational program
- Considers patient understanding

- Integrates different ways of teaching into delivery of care
- Creatively adapts teaching plan
- Partners with patients and families to identify, then meet, their learning needs

7. **Collaboration: Working with others (patient, family, health-care providers, colleagues, community) in a way that promotes and encourages each person's contributions. Involves interdisciplinary and interdisciplinary work with colleagues.**

- Participates in team meetings
- Able to provide/receive feedback
- Willing to be taught, coached, and/or mentored
- Open to team members' contributions
- Fine-tuning communication, delegation, and negotiation skills

- Seeks opportunities to teach, coach, mentor
- Facilitates active involvement and contributions of others
- Fully engaged in cooperative effort. Knows when to lead and follow.
- Proficient in providing/receiving feedback

8. Systems thinking: Appreciates the care environment from a perspective that recognizes the holistic interrelationships that exist within and across health-care settings

- Implements the change designed by others
- Operates on a micro level (local stance)
- Developing strategies to facilitate change
- Developing political savvy

- Operates on a macro level (global stance)
- Develops, integrates, and applies a variety of strategies that are driven by patient needs and strengths
- Possesses political savvy within complex system
- Able to evaluate system breakdown
- Orchestrates the environment and resources within and across health-care systems.

PES conducted critical incident interviews (see Box A.1) in the winter of 1995. The interviews were designed to elicit feedback from practicing nurses on a draft version of the patient and nurse characteristics. Those interviewed noted that (1) the nurse characteristics reflected current practice, (2) the patient-nurse match was often considered by charge nurses when assigning nurses to patients, and (3) the characteristics were critical in achieving desirable patient outcomes. Participants also helped the SME group identify areas that needed further clarification. The reviewers had difficulty differentiating team participation and systems management. Staff nurse reviewers commented that nurse managers, not staff nurses, managed systems and that systems management was an important dimension for the future but not part of current reality. Almost every nurse interviewed was either unfamiliar with or felt uncomfortable with the use of the word "agency." For most nurses, "agency" meant a place to hire per-diem nurses. Clinical inquiry was singled out as an important dimension that distinguishes nursing as a professional discipline. Participants commented that the educational role of the nurse was not present. Many stated that the environment or the hospital/institution directly affects whether and how nurses display the characteristics.

Box A.1. Critical Incident Interviews (CII)

After the SME group defined and described an initial draft of the patient and nurse characteristics, PES designed a validation process. The purpose of the CII was to verify the clarity and comprehensiveness of the patient characteristics and nurse competencies and to pilot test a review process.

The SME group developed "patient profiles" that resembled an expanded nurse-nurse patient report. Three levels of profiles (low, medium, and highly critical) were prepared, reflecting adult, pediatric, and neonatal practice.

The profiles were designed to reflect data that (1) would be available after caring for a patient for a single shift; (2) would be communicated to another nurse, considered competent, with about 1 year of experience; (3) would be necessary to adequately care for the patient for the first time. Profiles included both qualitative comments and flow sheet data. The following types of information were included in the patient profiles:

- Demographics

- Presenting problem

- How patient presented

- Course of illness

- Issues and concerns

- Risk analysis

- Systems review

- Review of the most recent shift (including flow sheet data)

- Current treatment

- Management of issues and concerns

- Likes/dislikes of the patient

- Information concerning family/significant others

- Summary statement

Each member of the SME group nominated three experienced nurses who worked in ambulatory care, acute care, and critical care. From this pool of nominees, 33 nurses reflecting a wide spectrum of experience, education, and geographical location were selected and interviewed.

Prior to the interview, participants were given the nurse characteristics and continua for review. In preparation for the interview, the participants were asked to review the materials and rate their colleagues using the nurse characteristics ratings. Participants were interviewed by telephone and asked to react to the nurse characteristics and their continua. They were also asked to complete a rating exercise that described the patient characteristics. Interviewer notes and ratings were reviewed for common themes and general concerns, and a comprehensive report was presented to the SME group and reviewed during the March 29-31, 1996, meeting.

Based upon the review, several refinements were made to the model. Agency was rephrased to advocacy/moral agency. Team management was redefined as collaboration. Systems management was rephrased to systems thinking. Numerous descriptors were added to the continuums of each dimension.

The outcomes think tank (see Table A.6) was convened March 1-2, 1996, in San Francisco. The goal of the meeting was to articulate "optimal patient outcomes" that one would expect to result from certified practice based on the reconceptualized model. The science of outcomes measurement, especially as it related to nursing, was in its infancy at the time. Thus the group was not charged with identifying concrete measures or methodologies, but rather a framework to help guide thinking and a future research agenda. At this meeting, the "Synthesis" Model was termed the "Synergy" Model. It was explained to the group that the dynamic interaction, or synergy, between patient needs and nurse characteristics results in optimal patient outcomes. After reviewing the SME work, Dr. Patricia Benner specifically recommended that the group consider making the role of nurse as educator explicit; thus, facilitator of learning was removed from each dimension and reset into its own category. The outcomes think tank agreed that:

1. Outcomes should be relevant and important to the patient and family;

2. Individual patients, individual nurses, teams, and systems mediate nursing's capacity to influence patient outcomes;

3. Patients and families are active participants in the care process, and accountability for achieving optimal patient outcomes is a shared responsibility among all members of the health-care team;

4. Outcomes can be generic or disease-specific; outcomes can also be patient-, system-, or population-based;

5. Outcomes can be short-term or long-term, so measurement should be strategic in importance and timing.

Table A.6. Outcomes Think Tank

Patricia Benner, RN, PhD
Martha A.Q. Curley, RN, MSN, CCRN
Marion Johnson, RN, PhD
Marguerite Kenny, RN, DNSc, FAAN
Benton Lutz, MDiv, EdS
Patricia Moloney-Harmon, RN, MS, CCRN
Alvin Tarlov, MD
Staff:
Melissa Biel, RN, MSN
Wanda Roberts Johanson, RN, MN
Cheri White, RN, MSN, CCRN

A framework for optimal patient outcomes was developed. Outcomes were viewed to occur at three levels: patient, caregiver, or system. Outcomes viewed from the patient's perspective included, but were not limited to: patient ratings of care, patient satisfaction, patient trust (of the nurse), patient comfort, patient behavioral/knowledge, patient functional change, and patient quality of life. Outcomes viewed from the nurse's perspective included, but were not limited to: the extent to which care/treatment objectives were met, nurse assessment/management of physiological changes, and the presence or absence of preventable complications. Outcomes viewed from the system's perspective included, but were not limited to recidivism, health-care costs, and resource utilization. Nursing outcomes specifically include the preventative activities that nurses participate in and how nurses create environments and safe passage for patients and their families.

In May 1996, Martha A.Q. Curley, chair of the AACN Certification Corporation board, was interviewed by Michael Villaire of *Critical Care Nurse,* which resulted in publication of "The Synergy Model of Certified Practice: Creating Safe Passage for Patients" (Villaire, 1996).

The evolution of the Synergy Model was reviewed along with nursing's unique contribution to patient outcomes: specifically, creating safe passage for patients and families. In the mid 1990s, nursing was experiencing major restructuring and reorganization. Curley noted that:

> Nursing is in a critical, tenuous state right now; it can either get buried and deskilled and very disempowered; or, it can assume major leadership,

say what it does, take ownership for what it does by describing it, and move it forward. This [Synergy] model gives people some ideas, some language, to describe the contributions of a professional nurse. We have the potential to triumph if we really focus on what our unique contributions to patients are, and if we define ourselves in relation to patients. If we put the patient as primary and we base our practices on the needs of patients and hold the patient as primary, we'll be successful. (Villaire, 1996, para. 49)

As part of the Study of Practice, in March 1997 a validation survey (see Chapter 14) was launched. More than 3,500 critical care and non-critical care nurses of adult, pediatric, and neonatal patients were invited to participate in the mailed survey. The 21-page study booklet contained employment and demographic information and three sections. The first section reviewed the patient characteristics and asked participants to rate their usual patient population on a scale from 1-5 on each of the eight patient characteristics. The second section reviewed the nurse characteristics, then asked participants to rate their nursing colleagues' (nurses with whom they worked) level of competence on a scale from 1-5 on each of the eight nurse characteristics. The third section presented three separate patient profiles reflecting varying levels of acuity. After reading each profile, participants were asked to rate each patient characteristic on a scale of 1-5, rate the patient's overall criticality, then estimate the ideal level of competence required of the nurse on a scale of 1-5 to best meet the patient's needs.

Approximately 24% of nurses who were invited to participate completed the survey. In summary, the Study of Practice results supported the Synergy Model. Study results indicated that (1) patient needs were described using all eight of the patient needs continua; (2) there was a gradual step-up in perceived acuity from subacute to acute to critically ill patients; (3) nursing competency required to met patient needs can be described using all eight of the nurse characteristics continua; and (4) more compromised patients required higher levels of nurse competency.

In May 1997, Curley submitted "Patient-Nurse Synergy: Optimizing Patient Outcomes" for publication in *American Journal of Critical Care Nursing*. The purpose of the paper was to present the major tenets of the Synergy Model: patient characteristics of concern to nursing, nurse competencies important to patients, and patient outcomes that result when patient characteristics and nurse competence are mutually enhancing. It was noted that the Synergy Model clearly articulated the essence of the patient-nurse relationship and was conceptually relevant to the entire nursing profession.

In June 1997, the SME group reviewed the results of the validation survey. The newly formed strategic think tank (see Table A.7) joined the SME group at its final meeting, as the group was charged with evaluating the education, experience, and examination requirements for the CCRN exam based on results of the survey data. The group recommended that the Synergy Model serve as the new conceptual model for the CCRN exam, that PES develop test specifications, and that the new CCRN tests be available for administration by June 1999. Members of the strategic think tank recommended that approximately 80% of the exam be based on clinical judgment, and the remaining 20% on knowledge and skills of "Professional Caring and Ethical Practice," which include clinical inquiry, response to diversity, advocacy/moral agency, caring practices, facilitation of learning, collaboration, and systems thinking.

Table A.7.   Strategic Think Tank Members

Martha A.Q. Curley, RN, MSN, CCRN
Barbara Gill, RN, MN
Mairead Hickey, RN, PhD
Pam Mancini, RN, MSN, CCRN
Nancy Molter, RN. MN, CCRN
Patricia Moloney-Harmon, RN, MS, CCRN
Kathleen Shurpin, RN, PhD, CS, ANP, OCN
Anne Wojner, RN, MSN, CCRN

Staff:
Melissa Biel, RN, MSN (Staff, AACN Certification Corporation)
Sandy Greenberg, PhD (PES)
Pat Muenzen, MA (PES)
I. Leon Smith, PhD (PES)

The group also discussed the Synergy Model as it related to clinical nurse specialist practice. The group agreed that the traditional role components of CNS practice—specifically, expert practitioner, educator, consultant, and researcher—could be better articulated using the eight nurse dimensions of the Synergy Model. The nurse dimensions are identical, but the continuum reflects master's-degree, clinical-expert level practice. The eight patient dimensions are also identical but require expansion to include the CNS scope of practice, which includes activities with patients, nursing staff, patient populations, and systems in which care is provided. Working with PES, the AACN Certification Corporation developed and validated nurse characteristics descriptions for CNS practice (Muenzen & Greenberg,

1998). Both organizations then worked together to develop and administer the CCNS certification program.

In June 1999, AACN Certification Corporation contracted with Berlin Sechrist Associates to conduct a scholarly critique of the Synergy Model. The certification corporation wanted to identify the Synergy Model's strengths and weaknesses and obtain recommendations for refinement. Members of the American Academy of Nursing with expertise in theory critique were invited to submit their curriculum vitae to AACN and indicate their interest in serving as a member of the Synergy Model Review Panel. Ten individuals were selected from 84 candidates; 9 completed their review. Sechrist, Berlin, & Biel (2000) developed the Synergy Model review instrument criteria and criterion components (see Chapter 15). Overall, reviewer comments were positive and encouraging, and it was recommended that AACN Certification Corporation support Synergy Model refinement, identify ways to support testing of the Synergy Model, and partner with other groups to identify the ability of the Synergy Model to address their practice.

From 2001 through 2004, PES worked with AACN Certification Corporation to conduct the most comprehensive study to date of critical care nursing practice using the Synergy Model as a guiding framework. In this recently completed study, the Synergy Model was used to encompass the work of critical care nurses from entry level through advanced practice.

This history was reviewed and validated by the following individuals:

Melissa Biel, RN, DPA

Sandra Greenberg, PhD

Wanda L. Johanson, RN, MN

Pat Hooper Kyriakidis, RN, PhD

Patricia M. Muenzen, MA

Bonnie J. Niebuhr, MS, RN, CAE

Gayle R. Whitman, RN, PhD, FAAN

References

Ahrens, T., Yancey, V., & Lollef, M. (2003). Improving family communication at end of life: Implication for length of stay in the intensive care unit and resource use. *American Journal of Critical Care, 12*(4), 317-323.

Alexander, J.S., Younger, R.E., Cohen, R.M., & Crawford, L.V. (1998). Effectiveness of a nurse-managed program for children with chronic asthma. *Journal of Pediatric Nursing, 3*(5), 312-317.

Alspach, J.G. (2000). From staff nurse to preceptor: A preceptor development program, instructor's manual (2nd ed.). Aliso Viejo, CA: American Association of Critical-Care Nurses.

Alspach, J.G. (2005, May 9). *Preceptor empowerment #101 and #102.* Mastery session presented at 2005 AACN National Teaching Institute & Critical Care Exposition, New Orleans, LA.

Alspach, J.G. (2006). Extending the Synergy Model to preceptorship: A preliminary proposal. *Critical Care Nurse, 26*(2), 10, 12, 14.

American Association of Colleges of Nursing. (1998). *The essentials of baccalaureate education for professional nursing practice.* Washington, DC: Author.

American Association of Critical-Care Nurses. (2003). Safeguarding the patient and the profession: The value of critical care nurse certification. *American Journal of Critical Care, 12*(2), 154-64.

American Association of Critical-Care Nurses. (2005). *AACN standards for establishing and sustaining healthy work environments: A journey to excellence.* Aliso Viejo, CA: Author.

American Association of Critical-Care Nurses Certification Corporation. (1995). Redefining nursing according to patients' and families' needs: An evolving concept. *AACN Clinical Issues, 6*(1), 153-156.

American Association of Critical-Care Nurses Certification Corporation. (2002a). *Safeguarding the patient and the profession: The value of critical care nurse certification.* Retrieved February 2, 2007, from http://www.aacn.org/AACN/mrkt.nsf/Files/CertWhitePaper/$file/CertWhitePaper.pdf

American Association of Critical-Care Nurses Certification Corporation. (2002b). *Competency level descriptors for nurse characteristics.* Aliso Viejo, CA: Author.

American Educational Research Association, American Psychological Association, and National Council on Measurement in Education. (1999). *Standards for educational and psychological testing.* American Psychological Association. Washington, D.C.

American Nurses Association. (2000). *Scope and standards of practice for nursing professional development.* Washington, DC: Author.

American Nurses Association. (2001). *Code of ethics for nurses with interpretive statements.* Washington, DC: Author.

American Nurses Association. (2003a). *Nursing's social policy statement* (2nd ed.). Washington, DC: Author.

American Nurses Association (2003b). *Scope and standards of pediatric nursing practice.* Silver Spring, MD: Author.

American Nurses Association. (2004a). *Nursing: Scope and standards of practice.* Silver Spring, MD: Author.

American Nurses Association. (2004b). *Scope and standards for nurse administrators* (2nd ed.). Washington, DC: Author.

American Nurses Credentialing Center. (2003). *Magnet Nursing Services Recognition Program for excellence in nursing services. Health care organization instructions and application process manual 2003-2004.* Washington, DC: Author.

American Nurses Credentialing Center. (2004). *Magnet Recognition Program recognizing excellence in nursing services, Application manual 2005*. Silver Spring, MD: Author.

Arford, P.H., & Zone-Smith, L. (2005). Organizational commitment to professional practice models. *Journal of Nursing Administration, 35*(10), 467-472.

Balasco, E.M., & Black, A.S. (1988). Advancing nursing practice: Description, recognition and reward. *Nursing Administration Quarterly, 12*(2), 52-62.

Barnum, B.S. (1998). *Nursing theory: Analysis, application, evaluation* (5th ed.). Philadelphia: Lippincott.

Benner, P. (1984). *From novice to expert: Excellence and power in clinical nursing practice*. Menlo Park, CA: Addison Wesley.

Benner, P., Hooper-Kyriakidis, P., & Stannard, D. (1999). *Clinical wisdom and interventions in critical care: A thinking-in-action approach*. Philadelphia: Saunders.

Benner, P., Tanner, C.A., & Chesla, C.A. (1996). *Expertise in nursing practice: Caring, clinical judgment, and ethics*. New York: Springer.

Bradley, D. (2006, October). *ASPIRE: A creative advancement program*. Paper presented at the ANCC 10th National Magnet Conference, Denver, CO.

Brewer, B.B. (2006). Is patient acuity a proxy for patient characteristics of the AACN Synergy Model for Patient Care? *Nursing Administration Quarterly, 30*(4), 351-357.

Brewer, B.B., Pacini, C., Triola, N., Wallace, M., & Wojner-Alexandrov, A.W. (2005). *AACN Synergy Model for Patient Care: The "patient side" of the model*. Paper presented May 2005 at the American Association of Critical-Care Nurses National Teaching Institute.

Brewer, B.B., Wojner-Alexandrov, A.W., Triola, N., Pacini, C., Cline, M., Rust, J.E., & Kerfoot, K. (2007). AACN Synergy Model's characteristics of patients: Psychometric analyses in a tertiary care health system. *American Journal of Critical Care, 16*, 156-165.

Brooten, D., Youngblut J.M., Brown, L., Finkler, S.A., Neff, D.F., & Madigan, E. (2001). A randomized trial of nurse specialist home care for women with high-risk pregnancies: Outcomes and costs. *American Journal of Managed Care, 7*(8), 793-803.

Centers for Disease Control and Prevention. (2002). Guidelines for the prevention of intravascular catheter-related infections. *Mortality and Morbidity Weekly Report, 52*(RR-10), 1-29.

Centers for Disease Control and Prevention. (2003). National nosocomial infections surveillance (NNIS) system report: Data summary from January 1992 through June 2003, issued August 2003. *American Journal of Infection Control, 31*(8), 481-498.

Clarke, S.P., & Aiken, L.H. (2003). Failure to rescue. *American Journal of Nursing, 7*(8), 793-803.

Clifford, J.C. (2004). The essence of practice. *Excellence in Nursing Knowledge, 1*, 1-2. Retrieved October 26, 2004, from http://www.nursingknowledge.org/Portal/main. aspx?pageid=3507&contentID=56410

Cohen, S.S., Crego, N., Cuming, R.G., & Smyth, M. (2002). The Synergy Model and the role of clinical nurse specialists in a multihospital system. *American Journal of Critical Care, 11*(5), 436-446.

Collins, J. (2001). *Good to great: Why some companies make the leap and others don't.* New York: Harper Business.

Collopy, K.S. (1999). The Synergy Model in practice. Advanced practice nurses guiding families through systems. *Critical Care Nurse, 19*(5), 80-85.

Council on Licensure, Enforcement, and Regulation and the National Organization for Competency Assurance. (1993). *Principles of fairness: An examining guide for credentialing boards.* Author. Lexington, KY.

Covey, S.R. (1999). *Habits of highly effective people.* Year in a Box Calendar. Indianapolis, IN: Ventures, Inc.

Cox, E. (2003). Synergy in practice: Caring for victims of intimate partner violence. *Critical Care Nursing Quarterly, 26*(4), 323-330.

Cox, M. (2004). Implementing the synergy model within a multi-hospital system. *Excellence in Nursing Knowledge.* Retrieved 12 October 2007 from http://www.nursing-knowledge.org/Portal/main.aspx?pageid=3507&ContentID=56449.

Curley, M.A.Q. (1996). The Synergy Model of certified practice: Creating safe passage for patients. Interview by Michael Villaire. *Critical Care Nurse, 16*(4), 94-99.

Curley, M.A.Q. (1997). Mutuality — an expression of nursing presence. *Journal of Pediatric Nursing, 12*(4), 1-6.

Curley, M.A. (1998). Patient-nurse synergy: Optimizing patients' outcomes. *American Journal of Critical Care, 7*(1), 64-72.

Curley M.A.Q. (2004). Synergy Model. *Excellence in Nursing Knowledge.* Retrieved September 25, 2007, from http://www.nursingknowledge.org/Portal/main.aspx?pageid=3508&ContentID=55889

Curley, M.A.Q., & Hayes, C. (2003, March). *Parents' perceptions of being cared for well.* Oral presentation at the meeting of the Eastern Nursing Research Society, 15th Annual Scientific Sessions, New Haven, CT.

Curley, M.A.Q., & Hickey, P.A. (2006). The Nightingale metrics: What nurses do to "put the patient in the best condition for nature to act upon them." *American Journal of Nursing, 106*(10), 66-70.

Czerwinski, S., Blastic, L., & Rice, B. (1999). The Synergy Model: Building a clinical advancement program. *Critical Care Nurse, 19*(4), 72-77.

Dana-Farber Cancer Institute. (n.d.). *Mission and values.* Retrieved October 1, 2007, from http://www.dana-farber.org/abo/mission/default.html

Deisch, P., Soukup, M., Adams, P., & Wild, M. (2000). Guided imagery replication study using coronary artery bypass graft patients. *Nursing Clinics of North America, 35*(2), 417-425.

DeVellis, R.F. (1991). *Scale development: Theory and applications.* Newbury Park, CA: Sage.

Dilorio, C., Price, M.E., & Becker, J.K. (2001). Neuroscience nurse internship program: The first decade. *Journal of Neuroscience Nursing, 33*(1), 42-52.

Doble, R.K., Curley, M.A.Q., Hession-Laband, E., Marino, B.L., & Shaw, S.M. (2000). The Synergy Model in practice. Using the Synergy Model to link nursing care to diagnosis-related groups. *Critical Care Nurse, 20*(3), 86-92.

Duggan, W. (2003). *The art of what works.* New York: McGraw Hill.

Durley, C.C. (2005). *The NOCA guide to understanding credentialing concepts.* White paper on credentialing (1-11). Retrieved February 2, 2007, from http://www.noca.org/members/CredentialingConcepts.pdf

Edwards, D.F. (1999). The Synergy Model: Linking patient needs to nurse competencies. *Critical Care Nurse, 19,* 88-90.

Fabrey, L. (1996). Basic psychometric principles. In A.H. Browning, A.C. Bugbee, & M.A. Mullins (Eds.), *Certification: A NOCA handbook* (pp. 1-40). Washington, DC: National Organization for Competency Assurance.

Fawcett, J. (1995). *Analysis and evaluation of conceptual models of nursing* (3rd ed.). Philadelphia: F.A. Davis.

Fawcett, J. (2005). *Contemporary nursing knowledge: Analysis and evaluation of nursing models and theories* (2nd ed.). Philadelphia: F.A. Davis.

Fulton, J.S. (2003). New view, same mission. *Clinical Nurse Specialist, 17*(3), 117-118.

Gerberding, J.L. (2002). Hospital-onset infections: A patient safety issue. *Annals of Internal Medicine, 137*(8), 665-670.

Giles, P.F., & Moran, V. (1989). Preceptor program evaluation demonstrates improved orientation. *Journal for Nurses in Staff Development, 5*(1),17-24.

Goleman, D. (1998). *Working with emotional intelligence.* New York: Bantam.

Green, D. (2006). A Synergy Model of nursing education. *Journal for Nurses in Staff Development, 22*(6), 277-283.

Greenleaf, R.K. (1996). *On becoming a servant leader.* San Francisco: Jossey-Bass.

Greenberg, S., Smith, I.L., & Curtin, J. (1991). An analysis. In A.H. Browning, A.C. Bugbee, & M.A. Mullins (Eds.), *Certification: A NOCA handbook* (pp. 41-66). Washington DC: National Organization for Competency Assurance.

Gul, R.B. & Boman, J.A. (2006). Concept mapping: A strategy for teaching and evaluation in nursing education. *Nurse Education in Practice, 6*, 199-206.

Hardin, S.R. (2004). Using the Synergy Model with undergraduate students. *Excellence in Nursing Knowledge, 1*, 1. Retrieved March 2, 2007, from www.nursingknowledge.org.

Hardin, S.R., & Kaplow, R. (2004). *Synergy for Clinical excellence: The AACN Synergy Model.* Sudbury, MA: Jones & Bartlett.

Henderson, V. (1960). *Basic principles of nursing care.* London: International Council of Nurses.

Hsu, L. (2004). Developing concept maps from problem-based learning scenario discussions. *Journal of Advanced Nursing, 48*(5), 510-518.

Hsu, L., & Hsieh, S. (2005). Concept maps as an assessment tool in a nursing course. *Journal of Professional Nursing, 21*(3), 141-149.

Joint Commission on Accreditation of Healthcare Organizations. (2004). *National patient safety goals.* Retrieved February 28, 2007, from www.jcaho.org

Joint Commission on Testing Practices. (1988). *The code of fair testing practices in education*. Author. Washington, D.C.

Kaplow, R. (2002). *Applying the Synergy Model to nursing: A definition and its implications for practice, research, and education*. New York: Macmillan.

Kaplow, R. (2003). AACN synergy model for patient care: A framework to optimize outcomes. *Critical Care Nurse*, (Suppl.), 27-30.

Kautz, D.D., Kuiper, R.A., Pesut, D.J., Knight-Brown, P., & Daneker, D. (2005). Promoting clinical reasoning in undergraduate nursing students: Application and evaluation of the outcome present state test (OPT) model of clinical reasoning. *International Journal of Nursing Education Scholarship, 2*(1), 1-19.

Kerfoot, K. (2001). The art of raising the bar. *Nursing Economics, 19*, 125-126.

Kerfoot, K., & Cox, M. (2005). The Synergy Model: The ultimate mentoring model. *Critical Care Nursing Clinics of North America, 17*, 109-112

Kerfoot, K.M., Lavandero, R., Cox, M., Triola, N., Pacini, C., & Hanson, M.D. (2006). Conceptual models and the nursing organization. *Nurse Leader, 4*(4), 20-26.

Koerner, J.G., & Karpiuk, K.L. (1994). *Implementing differentiated nursing practice, transformation by design*. Gaithersburg, MD: Aspen.

Kotter, J. (1995). Leading change: Why transformational efforts fail. *Harvard Business Review, 73*(2), 59-68.

Kramer, M., & Schmalenberg, C. (1988). Magnet hospitals, part I: Institutions of excellence. *The Journal of Nursing Administration, 18*(1), 13–24.

Kramer, M., & Schmalenberg, C. (1988). Magnet hospitals, part II: Institutions of excellence. *The Journal of Nursing Administration, 18*(2), 11–19.

Kuiper, R.A., & Pesut, D.J. (2004). Promoting cognitive and metacognitive reflective reasoning skills in nursing practice: Self-regulated learning theory. *Journal of Advanced Nursing, 45*(4), 381-391.

Manworren, R.C.B. (2000). Pediatric nurses' knowledge and attitudes survey regarding pain. *Pediatric Nursing, 26*(6), 610-614.

McClure, M., & Hinshaw, A.S. (2002). *Magnet hospitals revisited: Attraction and retention of professional nurses*. Washington, DC: American Nurses Publishing.

McIver, J.P., & Carmines, E.G. (1981). *Unidimensional scaling.* Newbury Park, CA: Sage.

McNeil, S.A., Foster, C.L., Hedderwick, S.A., & Kauffman, C.A. (2001). Effect of hand cleansing with antimicrobial soap or alcohol-based gel on microbial colonization of artificial fingernails worn by health care workers. *Clinical Infectious Diseases, 32*(3), 367-372.

Meleis, A.I. (1997). *Theoretical nursing: Development and progress* (3rd ed.). Philadelphia: Lippincott.

Micheli, A.J., & Modest, S. (1995). Peer review. *Nursing Clinics of North America, 30*(2), 197-209.

Mitchell, P.H., Ferketich, S., & Jennings, B.M. (1998). American Academy of Nursing expert panel on quality health care. *Image: Journal of Nursing Scholarship, 30*(1), 43-46.

Mitchell, P.H., Heinrich, J., Moritz, P., & Hinshaw, A.S. (1997). Outcome measures and care delivery systems. *Medical Care, 35*(11 Suppl.), Entire Issue.

Moloney-Harmon, P.A. (1999). The Synergy Model: Contemporary practice of the clinical nurse specialist. *Critical Care Nurse, 19*(2), 101-104.

Muenzen, P.M., & Greenberg, S. (1998). *Final report for phase 1 in the development of a certification examination program for clinical nurse specialists (CNSs): Role delineation study for CNSs caring for acute and critically ill patients.* New York: Professional Examination Service.

Muenzen, P.M., & Greenberg, S. (2004). Conduct of the study practice validation survey. *Excellence in Nursing Knowledge.* August/September 2004. Retrieved 17 October 2007 from http://www.nursingknowledge.org/Portal/main.aspx?pageid=3507&ContentID= 56412.

Muenzen, P.M., Greenberg, S., & Pirrol, K.A. (2004). *Final report of a comprehensive study of critical care nursing practice.* New York: Professional Examination Service.

Mullen, J. (2002). The Synergy Model as a framework for nursing rounds. *Critical Care Nurse, 22*(6), 66-68.

National Association of Clinical Nurse Specialists. (1998). *Statement on clinical nurse specialist practice and education.* Harrisburg, PA: Author.

National Association of Clinical Nurse Specialists. (2004). *Statement on clinical nurse specialist practice and education.* Harrisburg, PA: Author.

Niebuhr, B.S. (1993). Credentialing of critical care nurses. *AACN Clinical Issues in Critical Care Nursing, 4*(4), 611-616.

Nightingale, F. (1946). *Notes on nursing: What it is and what it is not.* (Conclusion). Philadelphia: J.B. Lippincott. (Original work published 1890).

Pacini, C.M. (2005). Synergy: A framework for leadership development and transformation. *Critical Care Nursing Clinics of North America, 17*(2), 113-119.

Pesut, D.J., & Herman, J. (1998). OPT: Transformation of nursing process for contemporary practice. *Nursing Outlook, 46,* 29-36.

Pesut, D.J., & Herman, J. (1999). *Clinical reasoning: The art and science of critical and creative thinking.* Albany, NY: Delmar Publishers.

Pew Health Professions Commission. (1998). *Strengthening consumer protection: Priorities for health care workforce regulation: Report of the Pew Health Professions Commission.* San Francisco: Author.

Philips, J. (2007). The patient safety CNS: A new role for an established systems expert. In P.R. Zuzelo (Ed.), *The clinical nurse specialist handbook* (pp. 304-342). Sudbury, MA: Jones and Bartlett.

Porter-O'Grady, T., & Malloch, K. (2003). *Quantum leadership: A textbook of new leadership.* Sudbury, MA: Jones and Bartlett.

Rouse, C.L. (in press). Advanced practice nursing: Defining the practice. *Perioperative Nursing Clinics.*

Schoonhoven, C.B. (1981). Problems with contingency theory: Testing assumptions hidden within the language of contingency "theory." *Adminstrative Science Quarterly, 26*(3), 349-377.

Sechrist, K.R., Berlin, L.E., & Biel, M. (2000). Overview of the theoretical review process. *Critical Care Nurse, 20*(1), 85-86.

Shea, G.P. (2001). *Medicine and business bridging the gap.* Gaithersburg, MD: Aspen.

Shimberg, B. (2000). The role that licensure plays in society. In C.G. Schoon & I.L. Smith (Eds.), *The licensure and certification mission: Legal, social, and political foundations* (pp. 145-163). New York: Professional Examination Services.

Silber, J.H., Williams, S.V., Krakauer, H., & Schwartz, J.S. (1992). Hospital and patient characteristics associated with death after surgery. A study of adverse occurrence and failure to rescue. *Medical Care, 30*(7), 615-629.

Silva, M.C., & Sorrell, J.M. (1992). Testing of nursing theory: Critique and philosophical expansion. *Advances in Nursing Science, 14*(4), 12-23.

Simpson, E., & Courtney, M. (2002). Critical thinking in nursing education: Literature review. *International Journal of Nursing Practice, 8*(2), 89-90.

Smith, A.R. (2006). Using the Synergy Model to provide spiritual nursing care in critical care settings. *Critical Care Nurse, 26*(4), 41-47.

Tanner, C.A., Benner P., Chesla, C., & Gordon, D.R. (1993). The phenomenology of knowing the patient. *Image: Journal of Nursing Scholarship, 25,* 273-280.

Tarlov, A.R. (1992). The coming influence of a social science perspective on medical education. *Academic medicine: Journal of the Association of American Medical Colleges, 67,* 724-731.

Titler, M.G. (2004). Understanding Synergy: The model from the perspective of a nurse scientist. *Excellence in Nursing Knowledge.* Retrieved February 17, 2007, from http://www.nursingknowledge.org/Portal/main.aspx?pageid=3507&ContentID=56400

United States Department of Labor. (1978). *Uniform guidelines on employee selection procedures.* Author. Washington, D.C.

Villaire, M. (1996). The Synergy Model of certified practice: Creating safe passage for patients. *Critical Care Nurse, 16*(4). Retrieved October 5, 2007, from http://www.aacn.org/certcorp/certcorp.nsf/edcfc72ba47aaa708825666b0064bdcf/c33607b44ed98b75882566d400035755?OpenDocument

Visintainer, M.A. (1986). The nature of knowledge and theory in Nursing. *Image: Journal of Nursing Scholarship, 18*(2), 32-38.

Walker, L.O., & Avant, K.C. (2005). *Strategies for theory construction in nursing* (4th ed.). Upper Saddle River, NJ: Pearson/Prentice Hall.

Watson, J. (2001). Theory of human caring. In M. Parker (Ed.), *Nursing Theories and Nursing Practice* (pp. 343-354). Philadelphia: F.A. Davis.

Wheeler, E.C. (1999). The effect of the clinical nurse specialist on patient outcomes. *Critical Care Nursing Clinics of North America, 11*(2), 269-275.

Wheeler, E.C. (2000). The CNS's impact on process and outcome of patients with total knee replacement. *Clinical Nurse Specialist, 14*(4), 159-169.

Willoughby, D., & Burroughs, D. (2001). A CNS-managed diabetes foot-care clinic: A descriptive survey of characteristics and foot-care behaviors of the patient population. *Clinical Nurse Specialist, 15*(2), 52-57.

Zara, A. (2000). The mission of the National Council of State Boards of Nuring. In C.G. Schoon & I.L. Smith (Eds.), *The licensure and certification mission: Legal, social, and political foundations* (pp. 189-193). New York: Professional Examination Services.

Zungolo, E. (2004). Faculty preparation: Is clinical specialization a benefit or a deterrent to quality nursing education? *Journal of Continuing Education in Nursing.* 2004 Jan-Feb;35(1):19-23.

Zuzelo, P. R. (2007). *The clinical nurse specialist handbook.* Sudbury, MA: Jones and Bartlett.

Additional Relevant Readings

American Association of Critical-Care Nurses. (2006). Nurse competencies and patient needs from the AACN Synergy Model for Patient Care.

Anonymous. (2003). Multihospital system adapts AACN synergy model. *Critical Care Nurse, 23*(5), 86-88.

Berke, W.J., & Ecklund, M.M. (2002). Keep pace with step-down care ... first article of a six-part series. *Nursing Management, 33*(2), 26-29.

Conn, V.S., Burks, K., Rantz, M., & Knudsen, K.S. (2002). Evidence-based practice for gerontological nursing. *Journal of Gerontological Nursing, 28*(2), 45-52.

Ecklund, M.M., & Stamps, D.C. (2002). The Synergy Model in practice. Promoting synergy in progressive care. *Critical Care Nurse, 22*(4), 60-67.

Hardin, S., & Hussey, L. (2001). The Synergy Model in practice. Clinical inquiry. *Critical Care Nurse, 21*(2), 88-91.

Hardin, S., & Hussey, L. (2003). Using the AACN Synergy Model. AACN Synergy Model for Patient Care case study of a CHF patient. *Critical Care Nurse, 23*(1), 73-76.

Hartigan, R.C. (2000). The Synergy Model in practice. Establishing criteria for 1:1 staffing ratios. *Critical Care Nurse, 20*(2), 112.

Hayes, C. (2000). The Synergy Model in practice. Strengthening nurses' moral agency. *Critical Care Nurse, 20*(5), 90-94.

Hoffman, L.J., & Gill, B. (2000). Beginning with the end in mind. *American Journal of Nursing, 00*(5), (Suppl.), 38-41, 47-50.

Kaplow, R. (2002). Applying the Synergy Model to nursing education. *Critical Care Nurse, 22*(3), 77-81.

Kanaskie, M.L. (2006). Mentoring—a staff retention tool. *Critical Care Nursing Quarterly, 29*(3), 248-52.

Kerfoot, K. (2001). On leadership. The leader as synergist. *Nursing Economics, 19*(1), 29-;30.

Lenburg, C.B. (1999). Redesigning expectations for initial and continuing competence for contemporary nursing practice. *Online Journal of Issues in Nursing, 30,* 35.

Markey, D.W. (2001). The Synergy Model in practice. Applying the Synergy Model: Clinical strategies. *Critical Care Nurse, 21*(3), 72-76.

Mick, D.J. (2000). Guest editorial. Folklore, personal preference, or research-based practice. *American Journal of Critical Care, 9*(1), 6-8.

Mick, D.J., & Ackerman, M.H. (2000). Advanced practice nursing. Advanced practice nursing role delineation in acute and critical care: Application of the Strong Model of Advanced Practice. *Heart & Lung: Journal of Acute & Critical Care, 29*(3), 210-221.

Mullen, J.E. (2002). The Synergy Model in practice. The Synergy Model as a framework for nursing rounds. *Critical Care Nurse, 22*(6), 66-68.

Pope, B.B. (2002). Critical care. The Synergy match-up. *Nursing Management, 33*(5), 38-39.

Pope, B.B. (2002). Working together to meet patient and family needs. *Critical Care, 32*(7), 6-7.

Rapala, K. (2005). Mentoring staff members as patient safety leaders: The Clarian Safe Passage Program. *Critical Care Nursing Clinics of North America, 17*(2), 121-126.

Rohde, D., & Moloney-Harmon, P.A. (2001). The Synergy Model in practice. Pediatric critical care nursing: Annie's story. *Critical Care Nurse, 21*(5), 66-68.

Small, B, & Moynihan, P. (1999). The Synergy Model in practice. The day the lights went out: One charge nurse's nightmare. *Critical Care Nurse, 19*(3), 79-82.

Stannard, D. (1999). The Synergy Model in practice. Being a good dance partner. *Critical Care Nurse, 19*(6), 86-87.

Index

A